Providing Support to Young People

Practitioners who participate in helping, supporting or advising young people, whatever their role or working context, need a model to inform their practice. This invaluable guide to making the most of helping relationships concentrates on the practicalities and explores how to structure the help practitioners give to young people.

Providing Support to Young People discusses the context for contemporary youth support work before moving on to the practical development of the helping skills and strategies required by a practitioner. Drawing on established and 'new' approaches in guidance, the book presents a model developed specifically for the current working context where helpers work holistically across agencies for the benefit of young people. This framework:

- provides a structure for effective face-to-face interactions with young people;
- has a number of beneficiaries: the young person being helped, the practitioner, the employer and the funding body;
- is flexible, allowing for the range of situations in which youth support workers may be working;
- stresses the need for the work to be collaborative with the full involvement of the young people concerned.

Complete with case studies and reflective exercises, this practical book will be invaluable to all those working in information, advice, guidance and youth support settings, whether giving first-in-line or intensive support to young people.

Hazel L. Reid is Head of the Centre for Career and Personal Development at Canterbury Christ Church University. **Alison J. Fielding** is a Senior Lecturer in the Centre for Career and Personal Development at Canterbury Christ Church University.

Providing Support to Young People

A guide to interviewing in helping relationships

Hazel L. Reid and Alison J. Fielding

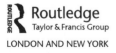 Routledge
Taylor & Francis Group

LONDON AND NEW YORK

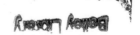

First published 2007
by Routledge
2 Park Square, Milton Park, Abingdon, Oxon OX14 4RN

Simultaneouly published in the USA and Canada
by Routledge
270 Madison Ave, New York NY 10016

Routledge is an imprint of the Taylor & Francis Group, an informa business

© 2007 Hazel L. Reid and Alison J. Fielding

Typeset in Sabon by BC Typesetting Ltd, Bristol
Printed and bound in Great Britain by
MPG Books Ltd, Bodmin

British Library Cataloguing in Publication Data
A catalogue record for this book is available from the British Library

Library of Congress Cataloging in Publication Data
Reid, Hazel L., 1951–
  Providing support to young people: a guide to interviewing in
helping relationships/Hazel L. Reid and Alison J. Fielding
     p. cm.
  Includes bibliographical references and index.
  ISBN 0–415–41960–3 (pbk.) – ISBN 0–415–41959–X (hardback)
1. Youth–Counseling of. 2. Social work with youth. 3. Interviewing in
social service. 4. Helping behavior. I. Fielding, Alison J., 1955– II. Title.
HV1421.R45 2007
  362.7–dc22
  2006034329

ISBN10: 0–415–41959–X (hbk)
ISBN10: 0–415–41960–3 (pbk)
ISBN10: 0–203–96210–9 (ebk)

ISBN13: 978–0–415–41959–8 (hbk)
ISBN13: 978–0–415–41960–4 (pbk)
ISBN13: 978–0–203–06210–7 (ebk)

#73993531

Contents

Foreword

Ever increasing numbers of young people are seeking advice, guidance and counselling. It remains as notoriously difficult as ever to quantify the effects, and in this sense the effectiveness, of these forms of support. However, provision responds not to demonstrable effects but to effective demand, which has risen, is still rising, and will continue to do so. The simple reason is that young people's life stage transitions have become more protracted and more complicated than in the past. This applies to education-to-work transitions. Spells in a variety of post-compulsory courses, training schemes and temporary jobs typically precede settling in an adult occupation (if settling ever happens). Housing and family transitions have also become more prolonged and complex. It is rare nowadays for a young couple to exit their parents' homes, to marry and establish a new family home all within a single day. It is now normal for young people to experience a series of sexual partnerships (typically between four and six) prior to marriage or cohabitation. Individuals are spending longer than in the past leading youth or young singles lifestyles, which means longer exposure to all the attendant risks. An outcome is that more of them seek specialist advice, more often than in the past, and for more varied reasons. They may feel unable to turn to parents or teachers. Doctors and clergy no longer claim to have all the answers. If they are asked, they may well feel ill-equipped to advise. They are among the sources of effective demand for more professional support for young people. So there are more and more professionals in education, health, housing, justice, careers, and youth and community services to whom young people with problems can be referred, or to whom young people self-refer, for 'support'.

This book is not a box of solutions. A plain fact of this matter is that there are rarely simple solutions to the problems of young people who are seeking professional help. It is the difficult cases that reach support workers' caseloads. Yet even without solutions to draw from their files, these professionals can always help, and this book explains how. It empowers support professionals by offering a toolkit – a template on how to proceed when a young person with a problem (very likely multiple problems) walks through the door. The toolkit is non-directive. It empowers support workers by enabling them to empower their clients to address their own problems. Whether the presented problem is about drugs, relationships, education or employment, support can usually start by encouraging clients to assess 'Where am I now?' then clarify 'Where would I like to be?' after which the question is 'How do I get there?' Working through these questions might take no more than a single session, or it might take weeks or months, but the template will fit most cases.

A client may decide, after due consideration, that he or she does not really want to get to 'b' but would prefer 'c', or that 'b' will be unattainable given the starting point, or that the road will prove too arduous. In other words, clients may well change their minds. Others will consolidate their original ideas. In either case an outcome of support should be a client with realisable aims that have been identified and adopted by, rather than presented to and imposed on, the client.

There can never be a guarantee that an 'action plan' will be fulfilled. Today's young people head into adult worlds that are full of uncertainties and risks. Planned destinations may disappear while young people are still in life stage transition. A relationship on which a person was relying may disintegrate through no fault of his or her own. New options constantly appear. The fully empowered client will be able to re-assess constantly 'Where am I?' 'Where do I want to be?' and 'How do I get there?' but in practice many become repeat presenters for guidance. Clients who return can be counted as successes, just like those who have no further need. The crunch test of effective guidance is whether clients who have further need return for more.

Up to now a common complaint from students who are training for youth support roles is that their courses are strong on theory (to which I confess to contributing) and relatively weak on the practicalities. Students learn about choice and opportunity, trait, developmental and other psychological and sociological theories. They learn about the need to be anti-oppressive, pro-justice, to respect cultural differences and to deliver equal opportunities. None of this tells them what to do when a client sits in the adjacent chair. This book will fill that gap. It will bolster youth support workers' confidence. They will know that they can always help even without solutions in their briefcases. This book is theory based but, like all the best theories, the theory in this book actually works because it is based on a wealth of experience in face-to-face guidance situations. Students will find that this book is not only interesting but also extremely useful. Their teachers will surely decide that the book is indispensable.

Ken Roberts
Professor of Sociology
University of Liverpool
August 2006

Acknowledgements

The authors wish to thank their colleague Jane Westergaard for her helpful comments on an early draft of the manuscript. Thanks also to Connexions Suffolk, whose interest in a model for 'intensive' personal advisers provided the impetus for the book.

Notes on authors

Hazel L. Reid is Head of the Centre for Career and Personal Development at Canterbury Christ Church University. She teaches on a range of undergraduate and postgraduate programmes, specialising in the area of career and guidance theory and career counselling skills. She serves on the Research Committee of the Institute of Career Guidance, is a member of the International Association of Educational and Vocational Guidance and of the Higher Education Academy. She has published widely and presented papers at national and international conferences. Her current research interests include support and supervision for youth support workers and developing narrative approaches for guidance practice.

Alison J. Fielding is a Senior Lecturer in the Centre for Career and Personal Development at Canterbury Christ Church University. A psychology graduate, she has been involved in training career guidance practitioners for many years, teaching on a range of programmes at undergraduate and postgraduate level. She has had extensive experience working with a number of Connexions Partnerships, in the training of personal advisers. She is engaged in research in the field of career guidance, current interests being young people's transitions into the labour market, inventing and re-inventing career identities and chance factors in the development of career narrative.

1   Introduction

Who is the book for – why do they need it?

> I thought what I needed to be effective was lots of information – knowledge about opportunities, agencies that could help and so on. I thought I would need to know all the answers and be able to tell a young person what to do, where to go – I'd be a fountain of knowledge! Since doing the course and learning the skills, I've realised that the most important thing is to listen and to find out about the client from their point of view. You have to do this to find out what they know – their story – before you can start to share your knowledge and support them effectively.

These are a student's comments during feedback from an assessed one-to-one interview on a training course for guidance practitioners. It was one of the 'best' interviews observed in the group that year, but that level of competence is not easy to attain and for the student it was hard won. Earlier in the year – let's call the student Sam – I observed an interview where Sam spent most of the time giving the young person information without achieving the level of engagement described above as 'the most important thing'. In the feedback of that earlier interview, Sam was rather pleased with the outcome and the assessor, Hazel, was not! My feedback focused on how she had overwhelmed the young person with information which, although not incorrect, was not based on an exploration of the young person's current situation, their interests, their concerns, their resources or their constraints.

Sam became very upset as she felt that her previous experience, as an employment and training adviser working with young people, meant that she knew how to interview. Her confidence was shaken and it took some weeks for her to 'unlearn' her previous approach and to adopt the young person-focused approach being taught: the approach described in this book. Sam had to change her style to acknowledge that a one-to-one interaction to support and engage a young person is not a formal information-giving interview, but neither is it just a cosy chat. It is not the same as talking to a friend but a professional conversation: what we describe as 'talking with a shared purpose'. The purpose being to support a young person in their decision making within their perception of what is important – not solely the helper's or the helping agency's view of what counts as important.

At the end of the course Sam demonstrated her new understanding in a series of very good interviews and in the feedback, following the final interview, made the comments that open this book. She also said, 'I was devastated by that feedback earlier in the year, but it was the best thing that could have happened. I know now the difference between giving information or advice and proper support and guidance. I get such good feedback from young people now – and they're the ones that really count!'

So who is this book for? We hope the book will become a recommended text for course tutors, trainers and practitioners working in the area of youth support work. This may include careers work, personal adviser work, youth and community work, youth justice work, social work, youth counselling and a range of other services for young people in, or connected to, education: for example education welfare, mentoring, teaching assistance, guidance and student support.

Practitioners and their trainers may be sited in higher education, further education, compulsory and private sectors of education, or within a range of youth support agencies, either state funded or voluntary. In addition to those studying for a professional qualification at a further or higher education institution, the book will be useful for those involved in professional or paraprofessional work-based learning. This may include S/NVQ courses in advice and guidance or learning and development support services and a range of foundation degrees reflecting cross-agency and partnership approaches to supporting young people and young people's services. It is intended to be an introductory reader, but it will also be useful for practitioners undertaking continuous professional development to review or update their knowledge and skills.

Before continuing we need to explain the terms used in the book. The generic term 'youth support worker' covers the intended audience, but is rather clumsy when used repeatedly. The title of 'personal adviser' is specific to England and to those practitioners working within Connexions services. We have used 'practitioner' or 'professional helper', or simply 'helper'. The word 'helper' does have problems as the need for help suggests an authoritarian view that 'disempowers' the individual. To counter this criticism, we will continue to emphasise the collaborative ethos of the work that underpins our approach. When describing one-to-one work with young people, we are aware also that the term 'interview' has formal connotations that may not resonate with the work: where appropriate we have used words such as intervention, interaction or meeting.

Moving on, why is the book needed now? Youth support workers working as 'personal advisers' may already have a professional qualification, for example from career guidance, youth work, social work or teaching, or be working towards a relevant qualification. If they are undergoing training then this book will be a useful resource. However, many youth support workers are engaged in providing individual support without specific training in an interview model that will help them to structure their interactions with young people. The book will enable those workers to develop such a model to make their practice more effective. This effectiveness has a number of beneficiaries: the young person being helped, the practitioner, the employer and the funding body. The model proposed, the Single Interaction Model, is flexible, allowing for the range of situations that youth support workers may encounter. But, it is an 'ideal' model that will need to be adapted within the 'messy' realities of practice (Schon 1983).

Numerous youth support workers who have completed training will be familiar with a model for structuring their work (e.g. Egan 2002) but, as indicated above, many of their colleagues will not. Personal advisers in the English Connexions services, whatever their background, will have undertaken specific training (CSNU 2003); however, that training does not include the development of a model for structuring one-to-one interventions with young people. Within the context of a government focus on youth issues, the book aims to fill a gap in the market by providing a text that is designed particularly for an increasing number of youth support workers. Feedback to us, the authors, from practitioners in the field suggests that other available texts, which focus on the traditional work of counsellors or careers advisers, are too broad in their scope and not relevant enough for the new working context. By comparison, this book is directly relevant to youth support workers, offering examples that focus on their concerns and practical experience. It provides the flexible framework that is needed for structuring the help given to young people within a resource-intensive, target-driven environment. This environment has become increasingly dependent on a broad and holistic approach to helping.

The context for holistic youth support services

The establishment of the Connexions service in England provided an opportunity to establish a collaborative service to support young people, paying particular attention to those who required additional support (SEU 1999). Although the Connexions model was not followed in the other 'home nations' in the UK, the issue of how to include young people 'on the margins' has been key in the re-structuring of youth support services. With the publication of *Every Child Matters* (DfES 2003) the sector for providing support to children and young people has grown in significance. The policy agenda resulting from ECM (*Every Child Matters*), and the subsequent *Youth Matters* Green Paper (DfES 2005), has highlighted the need for standards to be developed and evaluated in the provision of services. Practitioners engaged in helping, supporting or advising young people, whatever their role or working context, will need a recognised framework to structure their interactions with those young people.

Youth Matters moves towards a more socially grounded framework for helping young people within a partnership of resources at the local level, 'it is important that we integrate Connexions with a wider range of services at local level' (DfES 2005: para 39). This, along with the move to extend services based within schools, will give emphasis to the growing role of the paraprofessional within teaching and the voluntary sector. An interview model for structuring an effective helping relationship is as useful for the citizens' advice worker, the youth mentor, the student support assistant as it is for the youth worker, careers adviser or personal adviser.

As academics, educators and trainers, it is the experience of the authors that youth support services are aware of this need and are offering additional training to ensure standards are met and effective use of resources is achieved. Indeed, it is as a result of a request from a Connexions service that the model outlined in the book was developed. We, the authors, have worked for many years as trainers of guidance practitioners and have developed a successful model for one-to-one guidance interviews. With the expanded context for youth support work, the model (previously unpublished) has been adapted and extended and is now relevant to the range of initial training courses and practitioners cited. The book is intended, then, to provide a text that is relevant across disciplines, and for the continuing development of multi-agency and holistic services for young people.

Although aimed at the UK market, we hope the book will also have a wider appeal. Wherever services for young people are managed, there is a need to address the issues related to effective helping for those delivering the services. The cross-disciplinary nature of the structures adopted in England has reframed these issues: these are addressed in the way the model offered has been developed. With a global interest in the concept of inclusion, both economic and social, practitioners in other countries will, it is anticipated, find the material useful for their own working context.

What else is available?

It may seem strange to introduce other reading material at this point in the book, but we want to acknowledge some of the literature that has informed our approach. The existing core text for many professionals in the area of guidance, counselling and youth support work will be Egan's *The Skilled Helper* (2002). It is an excellent book: however, Egan's model is designed primarily for counselling relationships. *The Skilled Helper* is well written, regularly updated and full of useful examples, but may be too complex for situations where the practitioner is not involved in a sustained counselling relationship with a young person. Egan is particularly valuable for the experienced youth support worker: in other words Egan revisited, once you know what you are doing, becomes an illuminating read. The model used in this book is derived from Egan's three-stage model and draws significantly from his work, but adapts it to the context described earlier.

What else? Corfield (1995) has provided a good practical text for those wishing to develop their interview skills as career guidance practitioners. Although this has many practical examples the focus is on careers advisory work and does not extend to the current market for youth support services. Other texts include Culley and Bond (2004) who also draw on counselling models and apply these to a range of guidance and counselling activities. The book is easy to read and is written in accessible language and illustrated by useful examples. Although up-to-date, it is not written specifically for youth support work. Nelson-Jones (2005) provides another excellent text for a general counselling model.

Less practical but good for the academic underpinning of an interaction model are the following texts: Jayasinghe (2001), Kidd (1996) and Gothard *et al.* (2001). Besley (2002) offers a rich and challenging text on youth counselling, but this is more relevant for the experienced counsellor or academic and may prove too challenging for the novice practitioner. Similarly, there are numerous texts from North America and Australia from the career counselling sector, where the focus is on counselling, rather than the wider context of youth support work. These texts explore 'career theory', or how individuals make educational or vocational decisions and draw heavily on the disciplines of psychology and sociology.

To clarify, this book does not cover career, personal development or decision making theory: these are already provided for adequately in existing US and UK texts. This book concentrates on the practice of how to intervene in the process – how to structure the help practitioners give to young people when they engage, or need to engage, with a decision making process. In other words, talking with a shared purpose.

The style of writing in the book

Practitioners are involved in what is often euphemistically called 'busy practice'. They need to access and assimilate knowledge as they practice. Long 'probation' periods of training are, in many professional and para-professional contexts, replaced with a mix of training and learning in the workplace. Nevertheless in a context of constant policy change where practice must evolve rapidly, practitioners need underpinning knowledge as well as practical experience. The book sets out to balance the relationship between theory, policy and practice. We are aware of the need for critical engagement with the dictates of a policy approach that can lead to de-professionalisation via integration of services (see Watts 2006), but have not entered that discussion within this text.

So, whilst this book is underpinned by academic rigour, which is supported by references and theoretical understanding, its rationale is to provide access to the one-to-one interview model. In so doing it is written in an easy-to-read style and supported with practical examples, case studies, exercises and diagrams: all designed to help the reader to understand and apply the model to their practice. The 'isolated' individual reader will be able to develop their practice using the book, although the intention is that this becomes a text for use alongside others on initial, professional and paraprofessional training courses. Although the interview model can be used in other guidance sectors (for example, working with adults) we have kept the focus on the growing sector of working with young people: the examples of the model in practice will be targeted at this group.

The next section in this introductory chapter outlines the content of the book. Whether you are a novice practitioner, trainer or an experienced youth support worker reviewing your practice, we hope you will want to read it all! However, you can of course focus on particular chapters selected to support an area of your practice that you are currently developing or reviewing. The Single Interaction Model (SIM) is fundamental for understanding *Providing Support to Young People*: both the book and the practice. We introduce the model in chapter 2 but leave the detailed examination to the final chapter. There is logic in progressing through the book from chapters 1 to 7, but readers may decide to take a different approach and look at the detail of SIM earlier. The presentation of each chapter should make possible this type of flexible approach to the material.

Content overview

The book discusses the context for youth support services and defines what is meant by 'professional helping' and guidance. It takes the reader through a range of activities that can be described as 'helping' in youth support work and clarifies the role of the youth support worker. It explores the theoretical background of the model and considers the outcomes of professional and paraprofessional 'helping'. The book then moves from context to the practical development of the necessary helping skills and strategies required by the practitioner, in order to help the young person move forward in their thoughts and actions. It also makes reference to selected counselling models that have particular relevance for helping young people: which can be explored further beyond the confines of this book. The final chapter looks at the stages of the model in some depth. The work is referenced throughout to signpost the reader towards relevant additional reading and an annotated bibliography is offered at the end.

Now read on!

We have enjoyed putting this book together. The original unpublished material, entitled *Guidance Explored* and used with students over many years, has been updated a number of times. The opportunity to publish the material has led to further deletions, adaptations, enhancements, additions and a number of reviews before it was ready for wider dissemination. It is no longer the same material. We have welcomed the chance to reflect on our approach and to progress our teaching practice – all part of the very necessary process of our continuous professional development. We have had to rethink our approach to meet the needs of young people and their helpers working in a changing context. This new learning and development makes our work interesting and parallels the experience of practitioners. What was it Sam said?

> I've realised that the most important thing is to listen and to find out about the client from their point of view. You have to do this to find out what they know – their story – before you can start to share your knowledge and support them effectively.

Talking with a shared purpose, as a guidance approach, does not evolve from a 'fountain of knowledge': the purpose is to work collaboratively with a young person. We hope engaging with the material will help you with that collaborative work. So, now read on!

2 Helping
Definitions and purpose

Introduction

This chapter explores the nature of a professional helping relationship with young people, by considering some fairly fundamental questions: What do we mean by helping? How much helping? How do you structure that work? Later chapters cover different aspects of a helping model for one-to-one work, so that each part can be considered separately: this, we hope, will enable readers to make sense of the whole model.

Trying to explain the concept of a model for a professional helping relationship is rather like trying to tell someone how to drive a car – instructions are clarified if you are actually *in* the car. Like driving a car, 'helping' makes much more sense if you are actually involved, though it does seem at times that there is just too much happening at once to be clear about what is going on. This book should help to make things clearer: it is intended very much as a practitioner's guide. We will use the word 'helping' in the rest of the book to signify a 'professional helping relationship'. In using the term 'professional' we are referring to a formal relationship (i.e. governed by ethical codes of practice) between the helper and the young person, and we are not excluding practitioners who are viewed as para-professionals or volunteers.

When discussing practice we are also going to use 'we' rather than 'you', and we will avoid writing exclusively in the third person. Our decision to use 'we' is an attempt to be more inclusive, to place ourselves within the practice we advocate and to avoid telling 'you' what to do. This is not a conventional approach for a theoretical textbook, but, as discussed in the previous chapter, although we will ground the model in the literature we do want to focus on practice.

A model of helping

The Single Interaction Model (SIM) has been developed to reflect the current context for personal advisers and youth support workers. We have chosen to refer to it as an 'integrated' approach as this seems to offer a clearer picture of the nature of the model. Kidd (1996) explores, in some depth, the concepts of 'technical eclecticism' and 'theoretical integration' that underpin approaches to guidance work. In brief a technical and eclectic approach uses tools and strategies without, necessarily, understanding the theoretical concepts that underpin the model. An approach that is theoretically integrated does acknowledge and draw on the theoretical models that inform the related tools and strategies that a practitioner chooses to integrate within their practice. There are advantages and disadvantages of adopting either approach and these are discussed by Kidd. In this book we explore the concepts that underpin the model, which make it an integrated approach, but we wish to focus on *how* to use the model. Practitioners are, of course, free to explore a range of ways of working with young people, and to draw on 'what works' from their existing knowledge: this enables the flexible response we advocate in order to meet a young person's needs.

Approaches to helping have been informed by a number of theoretical models – for example, humanistic, behavioural, psychodynamic and multicultural, all of which can inform an integrated counselling approach. The approach in this model of helping has much in common with other models and draws on many sources, as the phrase 'integrated' implies; however, whilst noting the limitations, there is a clear emphasis on the humanistic approach in counselling. The work of Rogers (1951, 1961) and Egan (2002), informs many of the models used in the counselling field. The concepts have been adapted here for the context of working with young people, but are applicable to a wide range of non-therapeutic settings and 'clients'.

Egan uses the term 'The Skilled Helper', and in this introductory section we would like to borrow the term. The aim of our book is to help or enhance practitioners' abilities to become skilled helpers, working alongside the young people that require professional help and support. That help is *goal-orientated* and it is in the *action*, related to agreed goals, that helpers can reach *positive outcomes* in their work with (not for) young people.

The approach to helping in the Single Interaction Model is, like many others, based on a 'client-centred' approach, which we will call a 'young person-focused' approach. The approach is neither directive nor nondirective; instead it is 'facilitating' in that the helper, working alongside the young person, acts as a guide to help the young person make their own decisions in the context of their own lives. This collaborative approach, being young person-focused, is non-prescriptive but follows a flexible, yet time-bound, structure. The young person-focused approach, and the need for boundaries, is discussed in more detail in chapter 5.

Applying the model to a range of circumstances

The model of helping explained in this book seeks to demonstrate that the principles of effective helping, and the skills and strategies that can be used, apply equally to the wide range of contexts in which professional helpers find themselves operating: for example with colleagues and agencies with whom they network or refer young people to. In effect, the skills and strategies that are outlined in the book can apply in any situation where communication and interaction takes place. Although this book uses the model for one-to-one work, it can also be adapted for work with small groups of young people. The high level of interpersonal skills and knowledge that helpers need has application beyond direct work with young people. Anyone involved in a 'working with people' context, necessarily participates in a wide range of communication activities, which may or may not be directly involved with 'clients'. Therefore, the model of effective helping and helping skills that is presented in this book is equally appropriate for a variety of other 'purposeful' situations. For instance, it could include the activities of mentoring, coaching and counselling in a range of settings.

Helping relationships: definitions and purpose

We often talk about helping, and assume that the people we are talking to have the same ideas about what this means. However, as with other commonly used terms, we do not check with them that this is the case. A common understanding and definition of a helping relationship is needed to help overcome any confusion that may exist.

Our definition:

> *A helping relationship enables the young person to move towards their personal goals and to strengthen their ability to manage issues or problems in their lives. It is a collaborative relationship characterised by flexibility on the part of the professional helper in identifying and meeting the individual needs of the young person.*

In common with many professions, the skill and the knowledge base of helpers is wide ranging. These will vary according to the context and the purpose of the helping relationship. Nevertheless, much knowledge and many skills will be common, although the type and range of services for young people will vary from setting to setting, depending on the function of the agency or service and the role of the helper.

All of these services will be for individuals but some other services will aim to meet the needs of those seeking help within a group situation. In addition, professional helpers may sometimes undertake tasks on behalf of young people, depending on their level of need. The helping relationship encompasses a wide range of activities to assist young people to benefit from that relationship. The activities engaged in by the helper will be dependent on the specific needs of the young person or group and are discussed in the next chapter.

A helping relationship should be a learning process that is open and ongoing. The process is reflective as well as outward- and forward-looking. Helping can take place through a wide range of formal and informal situations. A number of factors will contribute directly and indirectly to a young person's progress within the helping relationship.

These ideas will be dealt with in more detail in later chapters. At various points, we will give definitions of different aspects of the model. These are intended to break up the concepts into more manageable elements and will be expanded upon in the appropriate sections. For convenience, these are in italic type.

The purpose of the helping relationship

Everyone seeks help at some time, and this usually involves some type of helping relationship. The difference for professional helpers is that we need to be clear about the intention of the helping relationship. Simply building a relationship and 'being there' for young people is not enough. We need to ensure that our help is focused on the needs of the young person and that together, within the helping relationship, we are moving on from the current situation. The young person needs to know what we can, and perhaps more importantly what we cannot, help with; what the expectations are within the helping relationship; what the benefits of getting involved might be and what the possible outcomes are. In short, the professional helper is engaging in a helping relationship with a young person for a purpose; that of 'moving the young person on' so that, ultimately, they no longer require the help of a professional.

By 'moving the person on' we mean helping them to progress, develop or move forward from the place they are when they seek help. That movement involves identifying what the young person views as a meaningful goal. That said, the degree of movement depends on the individual and their circumstances. For some, even after the intervention of the helper, they may not progress at this time, but hopefully will have clarified their thinking and have learnt from the process of engagement. Clearly, the time this takes will vary depending on the needs of the young person, and their ability and readiness to 'move on'. The basis of an effective helping relationship lies in helping young people to recognise their starting points (and these will be different for different young people), to decide on their goals and to move from the first to the second. The rest of this book sets out to show how this can be achieved.

One of the most important things about defining the helping relationship is that the definition we use in our work says something about what we, as professional helpers, are aiming to achieve. It helps us to understand the purpose of our work with young people. This in turn leads to our being able to establish whether we are actually providing the service we think we should – we can evaluate our work against the definition. We can then set out to improve the service we offer in the light of the evaluation, undertaken at the individual and organisational level.

Individual needs

Definition:

> 'Needs' are literally what people need help with. In simple terms, this is what the young person 'presents' to the professional helper (or another helper who may be a friend or relative) to help them to make changes and implement decisions.

For example:

- The young person might need help with deciding what action to take about some aspect of their life. Thus the need is for decision making skills.
- The young person may not term their needs in this way and it is likely that they will refer to their needs as wanting advice or simply as getting help, in non-specific ways.
- In addition to needs that the young person has identified, albeit in non-specific terms, they may have needs they are unaware or less aware of.

For instance, in order to make the decision, they may need to think about what they want as a result of the decision made. It may be that they can only do this effectively if they have a certain level of self-awareness. If they do not have this level of self-awareness then the first need is developing self-awareness, which they do not present explicitly to the helper. It is the helper's task to identify these unknown needs as well as the known needs and work with the young person to meet these, so that they can move forward. Egan (2002: 243) discusses this in some detail in *The Skilled Helper* in terms of the helper's role in assisting the client to identify their needs and wants: 'counselors help clients answer the following two commonsense but critical questions:

- What do you want?
  and
- What do you have to do to get what you want?'

A 'common sense' approach is particularly attractive to professional helpers, who often have limited time to work with individual young people. Of course, we cannot assume that one person's common sense is the same as another's and, although they cannot guarantee quality, the purpose of ethical codes of practice is to provide guidelines and standards for our work. Perhaps a better way of describing the approach would be to say that the model follows a 'natural' sequence of a) identifying an issue, b) exploring the options, and c) moving from goals to action. We will return to this later when we think about how this 'natural' model may or may not fit within a range of cultural contexts.

Identifying the individual needs of a young person may involve formal or informal processes, and will require some sort of assessment of the situation for the young person. At its simplest, this assessment of needs may involve the young person telling you what they think they require help with, and some discussion of this to ensure that you, as the helper, understand what they are saying. As we have seen, it is not always as straightforward as this, and we may have to engage in a more formal assessment. It may involve the drawing together of a range of information about the young person from a variety of sources, discussion of this information with the young person to help them understand it, recognising the implications, and agreeing priorities. We will consider this further in the next chapter.

In summary, young people have a range of needs, some of which they are aware of, and others which they are not. A young person may bring these to a professional helper, or other adults, with whom they can develop a helping relationship. They seek help (or are 'sent') to identify goals, make decisions and plan and implement action.

The helping process

Definition:

> *The stages through which the young person progresses so that they can identify and choose appropriate goals in order to manage change in their lives and to make and implement decisions.*

As the above definition suggests, professional helping is often an iterative process. Young people may want help over a considerable period of time, and this need may occur and re-occur throughout the time of their contact with professional helpers. The Single Interaction Model (SIM) presented in this book is informed by the work of Egan but is adapted for shorter time-bound interventions. Figure 2.1 places Egan and SIM side-by-side allowing us to compare the two models. Whether and how the Egan model or SIM is used, is likely to depend on the level of support a young person needs.

The helping process aims to assist a young person to move forward to their next step in relation to the changes they are dealing with and the decisions to be made. Whether they seek professional help or not, they will go through a process, a series of stages that will help them to become aware of opportunities, to consider alternatives, to recognise decisions to be made, to identify the changes and choices they can make and so forth. If they do not seek professional help they may rely on informal help; that is, advice from friends,

Egan three-stage model	Single Interaction Model
Stage 1 – current scenario	**Stage 1 – negotiating the contract and agreeing an agenda**
• Story: the young person explains current situation.	• Introductions are made and the purpose is shared.
• Blind spots: helping the young person to identify and be clear about problems and issues.	• Young person is helped to focus on their current situation and raise issues for discussion.
• Leverage: which are the most important issues to focus on during the remainder of the work?	• Objectives for the interaction are discussed and prioritised.
	• An agenda for the interaction is agreed.
Stage 2 – preferred scenario	**Stage 2 – developing issues and identifying goals**
• Possibilities: helping the young person to identify what they want and if it is possible.	• The young person is helped to explore the issues in greater depth.
• Agenda: translating possibilities into realistic goals.	• Possible options for the future are discussed.
• Commitment: testing out the motivation, considering the difficulties and choosing the goals.	• Through discussion, sharing of information and evaluation of possible options, realistic goals are identified.
Stage 3 – getting there	**Stage 3 – designing, planning and implementing action**
• Strategies: helping the young person to consider strategies for action.	• Identifying possible courses of action.
• Best fit: which strategy is going to be most appropriate for this young person?	• Discussing and evaluating the benefits of particular courses of action.
• Plan: turning strategies into a concrete plan for action.	• Agreeing specific action to be carried out.
Stages completed over a period of time, but each interaction has a beginning (Stage 1), middle (Stage 2) and end (Stage 3).	*All three stages completed in a single interaction.*

Figure 2.1 A comparison of Egan and SIM.

family or other care-givers. They may also depend on events and experiences to inform and shape decisions, choices and outcomes. Alternatively, they may seek help and advice from a professional. That said, seeking professional help will not necessarily replace the informal advice from friends and relatives, but will add to the help that is available to them as they make their 'journey' from 'where they are now' to 'where they would like to be' at some point in the future.

It is important for helpers to recognise and acknowledge that informal help happens, and will continue to happen alongside any assistance they may offer young people in their role as a professional helper. Support offered by practitioners does not operate in isolation from informal help and the processes that this includes. Informal help will have a value for the young person and an impact whether positive or negative. Acknowledging the importance of the social context for the young person is fundamental for effective helping: helping which ignores the 'world view' of the young person is unlikely to make a difference. How a young person constructs meaning in their lives cannot be ignored or dismissed in the rush to find solutions to help them 'move on'. Working collaboratively, alongside the young person, means understanding the client's story and helping them to script a new story (Reid 2002). However, this does mean challenging 'unrealistic' (too high or too low) aspirations, working towards goals and clarifying and taking action, but these are advanced skills that the helper needs to use within a structured process. The ultimate goal of helping is that the young person will learn from the process and be enabled to help themselves, but through the process of talking with a shared purpose.

For some young people, professional helpers will need to advocate on their behalf, but will be mindful that they are trying to develop the young person's ability to act independently. The role of the helper here is to provide the scaffolding to support the young person in the process of learning how to move forward and construct their own future (Bassot 2003).

The stages of the helping process

We have described the helping process as something that enables the client to move forward in some way. This moving forward necessarily spans a period of time, which may be difficult to specify, but a period of time that will be constrained by the helping contract established between the young person, the helper and the helping agency. When snap decisions are made on impulse without any thinking time, it is unlikely that participation in anything that might be termed a *structured* helping process has taken place. Figure 2.2 depicts that process of engagement in a flow chart, to help us think about that overall structure for work with a range of young people. But, it is offered as a tool to think with: a guide rather than a 'prescription'.

Practitioners need to be aware of and use these processes of moving forward in order to be effective in the help that they give. That said, the work is not as linear as any structure or flow chart may imply. One of the key things to recognise is that young people seeking help, or 'sent' for help, will be at different stages in the process when they meet an adviser or provider of helping services. Much of the literature on the process of choice and decision making tends to imply that people present themselves at the beginning of the helping process and will, therefore, need help through each stage. In practice people are likely to present themselves at the point at which they are either stuck or confused, or aware of an agency that seems relevant to their needs. Yes, some will present themselves at the beginning in that they

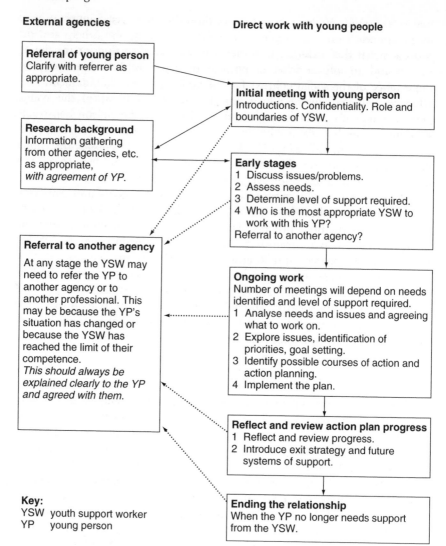

External agencies   **Direct work with young people**

Referral of young person
Clarify with referrer as
appropriate.

Initial meeting with young person
Introductions. Confidentiality. Role and
boundaries of YSW.

Research background
Information gathering
from other agencies, etc.
as appropriate,
with agreement of YP.

Early stages
1 Discuss issues/problems.
2 Assess needs.
3 Determine level of support required.
4 Who is the most appropriate YSW to
    work with this YP?
Referral to another agency?

Referral to another agency
At any stage the YSW may
need to refer the YP to
another agency or to
another professional. This
may be because the YP's
situation has changed or
because the YSW has
reached the limit of their
competence.
*This should always be
explained clearly to the YP
and agreed with them.*

Ongoing work
Number of meetings will depend on needs
identified and level of support required.
1 Analyse needs and issues and agreeing
    what to work on.
2 Explore issues, identification of
    priorities, goal setting.
3 Identify possible courses of action and
    action planning.
4 Implement the plan.

Reflect and review action plan progress
1 Reflect and review progress.
2 Introduce exit strategy and future
    systems of support.

Key:
YSW   youth support worker
YP   young person

Ending the relationship
When the YP no longer needs support
from the YSW.

Figure 2.2 The process of engagement.

have just begun to consider an idea; had thoughts about change, or have just
been plunged into some sort of crisis or change involuntarily. Equally, a
number will present themselves to helpers at a much later stage in an attempt
to make sense of any changes, choices and decisions that are affecting them.

An added dimension of the work for professional helpers is that they will
be, in many cases, working with young people who are not self-referred.
Working alongside young people who may resist the help on offer, can
add another layer of difficulty: this book will refer to this complexity as we
progress through the chapters.

How far along a young person is in the process of assessing their own situation and identifying suitable outcomes, will differ widely and depend upon a number of factors. An early task for the practitioner is to assess where the young person 'is at', in terms of the stages of the helping process, so that they can provide the help that is most relevant for that stage without dismissing what the young person has already 'sorted' for themselves. This careful approach avoids moving on too quickly when there are issues still to be dealt with.

Effective helping processes

In order to help young people in a positive way, practitioners need excellent interpersonal skills, and knowledge of what makes one-to-one work with young people valuable and effective for the individual concerned. It is unlikely that many young people will be able to move through the whole helping process in the space of one meeting. Some young people may need a series of meetings with professional helpers in order to meet all their 'helping needs'; whilst dealing with and moving forward towards the changes and decisions they wish to make.

Returning to the helping process as a series of stages that the young person moves through, we will now move on to identify the different stages that make up the whole process. What we present here is a three-stage progressive model that is adapted from Egan. The outline that follows is a brief synopsis of the stages (you can of course explore the detail of the Single Interaction Model (SIM) by reading chapter 7 next). Perhaps a note of emphasis is needed here. SIM provides a framework for practitioners to structure their one-to-one work, but it is primarily a model to help the young person to progress. In other words it serves both parties and enhances the collaborative working partnership that is its aim. In the outline of the model that follows we have tried to link the stage that the young person 'is at' together with an outline of where the helper fits into the process.

Stage 1 – current scenario (Egan 2002)
Negotiating the contract and agreeing an agenda
(Single Interaction Model – SIM)

At this opening stage the young person is helped to assess their current situation. This may include an assessment of their current thinking in relation to future plans (these may be educational or vocational or related to other needs). It will include an opportunity for the young person to tell their own story, in other words 'where they are at the moment'.

The practitioner will help the young person to identify their helping needs and consider ways in which these can be met. Depending on where the young person is in their thinking, the practitioner may help with the following as appropriate:

- Self-assessment and awareness; identification of possibilities and options; identifying current knowledge of opportunities and adding to this; decision making skills; referral and advocacy.

It is important that enough time is given to Stage 1 of the helping process, particularly if the young person is in any way resistant, confused, lacking in knowledge or understanding of the choices available to them, or unrealistic about what they are able to do or achieve. The helper needs to move at the young person's pace and in line with the young person's needs in order to move smoothly to Stage 2.

With some young people who require intensive support, it may take several sessions of rapport and trust building to achieve an agenda at the end of Stage 1: an agenda that clarifies the areas for future exploration and action. That said, each meeting will have a structure: a beginning – Stage 1, a middle – Stage 2 and an end – Stage 3 (Culley and Bond 2004).

Stage 2 – preferred scenario (Egan 2002)
Developing issues and identifying goals (SIM)

At this stage in the process the young person is ready to explore and identify possible future goals that are appropriate for them as individuals. Goals are not just what the young person wants to achieve in overall terms. Some goals may be targets of achievement, signposts or specific steps that pave the way for the future large or final goal. For some young people requiring intensive support, achieving small short-term goals can engender a sense of agency, an ability to make a difference in their own lives, and may be all that can be achieved for the present. But, this success is motivating and can provide a 'springboard' where, together, the helper and young person can move towards larger and long-term goals in and for the future.

So, in Stage 2 the young person and helper work together to identify the range of possible goals in order to help the young person choose those that are most appropriate and relevant, in relation to their values, abilities, aspirations, resources, context and needs.

Again, the helper and young person should not move on to the next stage until explicit goals have been agreed. Both the young person and helper need to be clear about what they are trying to achieve before moving on. Of course, when working intensively with a young person over a period of time those goals will change, but progress and positive outcomes will be the aim.

Stage 3 – getting there (Egan 2002)
Designing, planning and implementing action (SIM)

This is the stage at which the young person and helper look at what action could be taken, to enable the young person to achieve the goals that have been identified in Stage 2 of the process.

Together they can identify a range of actions that could be taken to get the young person to where they want to be. From this the young person can select the action that seems most appropriate and within their capabilities for the goals (small or large, short-term or long-term) that have been agreed. It is likely that for some young people, who require the helper to advocate on their behalf, some agreed action will also be undertaken by the helper. Together the helper and young person will formulate an action plan, and, depending on the circumstances, this may or may not be written down. The helper may need to assist with and follow up the implementation of the action plan, which might include the identification of further action. This will certainly be the case where a young person needs on-going help. Figure 2.3 depicts the three stages as diamonds to indicate the process of *opening up* the discussion *then focusing*: moving from *the possible* to *the specific*, at each stage.

Helping is not a linear process

Although the Single Interaction Model is presented in three discrete stages, young people do not necessarily progress through each stage in a linear fashion. If there are a number of issues to be dealt with, or where trust and rapport need to be built over a period of time, a young person might be taken through one or two of these fairly directly. Other issues may stay at Stage 1 for a longer period of time, to be dealt with at a later date.

In addition, the extent to which the whole process is completed will vary from young person to young person. Some may want help with initial exploration and clarification (Stage 1), then feel quite confident to sort out their goal setting and action for themselves. Whilst others may present themselves more or less at the goal setting stage (Stage 2) and need some help with this and action planning. Where you start will depend on the young person's needs and how confident they feel about sorting things out for themselves. The practitioner needs to be ready to help and build confidence for young people who need extra or intensive support. This enabling process may or may not include advocacy, depending on the readiness of the young person to act independently.

The length of time spent on any one stage of the process will depend on the young person's needs and the amount of time the helper is able to commit to the work. The latter will depend on whether the young person requires minimal, additional or intensive support. That assessment of need will be a diagnostic task that takes place before more detailed help can be planned and implemented. The assessment will want to consider a range of factors that may impact on the young person's ability to work independently on their future needs. A well known model of assessing 'needs' is provided by Maslow.

The starting point for Maslow's (1987) theory of motivation and personality is that there are human needs and motivations which are common to us

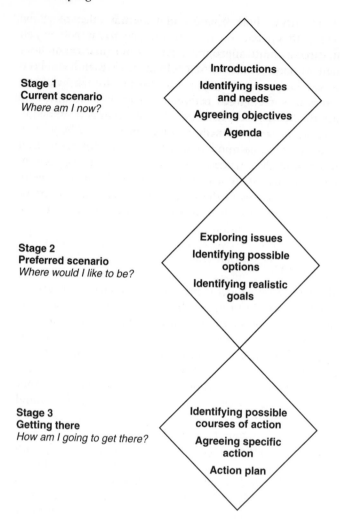

Stage 1
Current scenario
Where am I now?

Introductions

Identifying issues
and needs

Agreeing objectives

Agenda

Stage 2
Preferred scenario
Where would I like to be?

Exploring issues

Identifying possible
options

Identifying realistic
goals

Stage 3
Getting there
How am I going to get there?

Identifying possible
courses of action

Agreeing specific
action

Action plan

Figure 2.3 The three-stage model.

all, and which can be seen to follow a pattern as each need is satisfied. Maslow describes this as a 'hierarchy of needs'. At the most basic level, there are physiological needs – the essential requirements which must be satisfied if we are to survive, such as hunger or thirst. Once basic needs are satisfied, others emerge, which in turn lead to further needs and so on. Specifically, once the physiological needs are satisfied more social requirements, termed safety needs and encompassing security, stability, dependency, protection, the need for structure and so on, will emerge. Following the satisfaction of the safety requirements, love, affection and belongingness needs emerge. These involve both giving and receiving affection. Next, esteem needs emerge, the satisfaction of these leading to feelings of self-confidence, worth, capability and adequacy. Finally, self-actualization needs emerge, and meeting these results in self-fulfilment and the ability to become what one is capable of becoming. One of the key things about Maslow's theory is that is recognizes the relationship and interaction of the individual with society. It is this which enables us to look at Maslow's theory in relation to the work we do with young people.

Figure 2.4, based on an adaptation of Maslow's Hierarchy of Needs (1987), offers a framework for making that assessment and suggests the level of engagement that may be appropriate (with the emphasis here on 'suggests'). In addition, the notion of the young person's autonomy (ability to think and act for themself) is shown as a direct contrast to the level of need and probable level of intervention required.

For some young people, one or two sessions with a personal adviser or youth support worker may be all that is needed and all three stages of the model can be achieved in one meeting. Figure 2.1 offers a comparison between Egan's three stage approach that is developed over a number of sessions, and our adaptation – the Single Interaction Model (SIM) – for use within a single session or where intensive support is not, or is no longer, required. Linking the figures 2.1 and 2.4 we can see that the approach for helping young people who require less intensive help and who would benefit from one interview would be the Single Interaction Model (SIM). Conversely, those requiring additional or intensive support would benefit from an approach that follows the Egan model. That said, it is worth repeating that any 'engagement' can still follow a beginning,

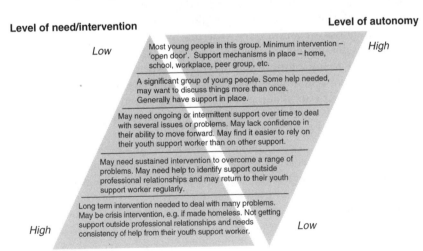

Figure 2.4 Assessment of need (based on Maslow 1987).

middle and end structure; in other words, SIM can be used for separate sessions. For example in the case study that follows, a young person in an immediate need for housing should still be fully involved in the decision making process of accessing help for their problem, even when the helper has to act quickly and is advocating on their behalf. The aim is that the interaction retains the ethos of talking with a shared purpose.

Andy: a crisis interview

Andy arrives at the centre needing to see someone immediately. He has just become homeless and has nowhere to stay tonight and no money. As the duty helper you meet Andy and move to an interview room. It is clear that he is distressed and you recognise that his immediate need is to be reassured that you will be able to help him, or if not can put him in touch with people who can. However, you want to build a relationship with Andy so that you can help him beyond this immediate crisis. Rather than spring into action at this point, making phone calls and so on whilst Andy sits and waits, having reassured him that you will be able to help, you spend a little time building rapport and trust. What do you do?

   You make sure he is comfortable in the room and check you are using his preferred name and that the details you have are correct – you explain why you are doing this. You clarify that he understands your role and how you can help today (he probably needs to hear again that you are going to help with the crisis) and you introduce the idea that you can work together beyond today. You are likely to want to discuss confidentiality at this point. You want to be clear about what his expectations are and you try to do this by asking him, before clarifying what is possible in the meeting today. You will want to give Andy an opportunity to say a little about his current situation (his story) so that you both have a shared understanding of what has happened. Having that shared understanding you will want to agree with Andy what needs to be done. Although Andy hopes you have the power to make a difference you still want to ensure you are not imposing your agenda on him.

   In the short time you have today (say, 20–30 minutes) you discuss the way forward. For example:

What are the options?
Who can help?
How can they help?
How does this fit with Andy's views about what needs to happen and how?

You are trying to keep Andy involved and are sharing information with him rather than deciding for him (albeit using your knowledge and experience).

Clear about the preferred options, you move to discussing action:

What needs to happen now?
What do you need to do as the helper?
What does Andy need to do?
What will help to make this action effective – for both of you?
What might get in the way?
So, what steps do you both agree?
When will you do it? In this case the 'when' will be now and later today.

Having engaged in a collaborative process, which did not place Andy in a passive position there is a good chance that rapport and trust has been built. Your long-term goal is to get Andy to return for further help once his immediate need is met. Part of the agreed action will be that Andy books an appointment (at the centre or elsewhere) or 'drops in' to see you again. And now you can leap into action, no doubt advocating on Andy's behalf!

1 So how does this 'case' fit with the Single Interaction Model?
2 How is it different from an immediate action response – what are the benefits of the SIM approach?
3 Can you think of an incident from your own experience or observation of practice that would benefit from this approach?

There are other models for helping the young person move forward that can be considered. Some of these may be derived from decision making theory, motivation theory, models for managing transitions or models for empowering young people. They can be found in literature relating to psychology, sociology, economics, counselling, work organisation and change, communication theory, learning theory or vocational choice and decision making. Some are referred to in later chapters: all have relevance, yet cannot be discussed in detail within the aims and limits of this book. As part of continuous professional development, a practitioner will develop their model, incorporating other knowledge from their own experience and alternative models and approaches. The references in the text will identify literature you may already be familiar with or want to explore. In addition, at the end of the book we have offered an annotated list for further reading.

Letting go

Professional helpers must also be ready to 'let go' of young people who feel capable and ready to manage things for themselves. We have to remember that we want to enable the young person to act independently and that they have the right to refuse our help. Of course some young people, despite our very best efforts, may not achieve independence; in these circumstances it is vital that we acknowledge the limits of our ability to help in a time-bound relationship. Such issues need to be brought to supervision to ensure best practice for those that are being helped, as well as to ensure the practitioner's well-being. If the practitioner's well-being is not addressed it is likely that work with 'clients' will not be effective and may even be detrimental (Reid 2006). Having a framework to structure the work can help both the practitioner and the young person to retain a sense of direction and shared purpose, even when the forward movement is minimal or slow.

Summary

In this chapter we have considered what we mean by a helping relationship. We have offered a definition of the term and also clarified what we mean by individual needs in the helping process. Two helping models have been introduced and discussed briefly, and a case study was included to show how the structure can be utilised for brief interactions. Diagrams were included in the chapter to give an overview of the process and to suggest how we might approach a diagnosis of how to use the 'helping' time available, where time is constrained by the organisational resources available. The skills involved will be looked at later; before that the next chapter will consider the range of activities that define a helping relationship.

3 Activities within the helping relationship

Introduction

This chapter continues to define helping by looking at the range of activities aimed at meeting the needs of those seeking help from a youth support worker. These activities were first explored in a paper produced by UDACE (the Unit for the Development of Adult and Continuing Education) in 1986. The definitions offered by UDACE were recognised as a significant step forward in trying to establish what is happening within a guidance or helping relationship. The seven activities identified in the paper formed a basis for subsequent explorations of helping relationships in other contexts. Not all of the activities will be appropriate all of the time. The activities engaged in by the helper and the young person will be dependent on the specific needs of the young person. We are making a distinction here between helping activities and helping or counselling skills; the latter are explored in chapter 6.

Helping activities

Definition:

> *Activities of helping are what helpers do (usually in conjunction with the young person) to help young people achieve positive outcomes and, therefore, have their needs met.*

For example, if the young person's need is for decision making, then we may employ a range of helping activities to assist this process. 'Enabling' (see below) is likely to be an appropriate helping activity in this instance, in that we can provide the young person with an opportunity to develop decision making skills and knowledge of the decision making process. We may also use 'advising' skills (see below) to help the young person to interpret information and choices, in order to work towards an appropriate decision.

These 'activities of helping' form part of the professional helper's 'toolkit' that they can use in order to meet the needs of young people. These activities are used together with helping skills in a variety of ways to achieve positive outcomes for the young person. Different models of helping describe these activities in slightly different ways: some give more emphasis to particular elements, depending on the context to which they refer. Some of these activities will form part of one-to-one helping discussions, as well as the wider range of interactions and tasks that make up the whole helping process. It may be helpful to offer a further point of clarification here: the Single Interaction Model is the framework that can help to structure the work – the activities described below may take place within an interaction with a young person or outside of an individual session. Indeed although the action should be agreed with the young person they may not always be present when you are; for example, advocating or networking.

From the original activities identified by UDACE in 1986, we have developed the following list to fit the context of professional helpers working with young people. In our attempt to define professional helping we need to separate aspects of the work: this fragments what is, in practice, an integrated process.

The activities of helping are as follows:

INFORMING   Providing information about opportunities, services, products, assistance and related support facilities available, without any discussion of the relative merits of alternatives for particular young people.

ADVISING   Helping young people to interpret information. This may also include helping the young person to choose the most appropriate option, service, etc. To benefit from advice, the young person must already have a fairly clear idea of what their needs are.

COUNSELLING   Working with young people to help them discover, clarify, assess and understand their needs and the possible ways of meeting these. This involves using counselling skills in the helping relationship.

ASSESSING   Helping young people to obtain a better understanding of their abilities and aptitudes, as they may relate to either personal, social, educational or career development, or the management of change in their lives. This is in order to enable them to make sound judgements about the appropriateness of particular courses of action. Such assessment may involve a range of methods, informal or formal.

ENABLING   Supporting young people when dealing with agencies, providers of products, services, education, training, employment and so on, in order to achieve positive outcomes and goals.

ADVOCATING   Speaking on behalf of young people for whom there may be barriers to access, whether individuals or groups, negotiating directly with institutions, agencies, or other professionals.

FEEDING BACK   Helping young people to evaluate their progress, and to recognise the things they need to do, and things they may need to change about themselves. Helping young people to take responsibility for themselves through greater self-awareness.

NETWORKING   Building relationships with other agencies and professionals in order to access a wider range of services or resources to meet the needs of young people. Referring young people, with their consent, to appropriate provision within other agencies.

REFERRING   Agreeing appropriate alternative provision with young people, when the professional helper has reached the boundaries of their own competence, and enabling young people to access this provision.

In practice all these activities are closely interrelated. Part of the skill of the professional helper is knowing when advising is the appropriate activity rather than providing information. So, for example, the choice of what information to present to a young person, and how to do so, involves some assessment of that young person, whether or not this is done consciously. In the same way, the 'confidence-building' role of the enabler often requires the use of counselling skills. It is also clear that effective referrals depend on the helper having a well-established network of other individuals and agencies to work with in order to meet the needs of young people.

It is worth considering the activities in more detail, and in what follows we have provided some examples to illustrate the different ways the activities can be used.

Informing

In work with young people, there is generally an emphasis on the need for clear and impartial information, and this is very important for enabling young people to make effective choices and to move on. The involvement of young people in identifying the group's likely information needs is helpful: the effectiveness of this approach is supported by research that has investigated the contribution of young people in focus groups which look at local provision. For example:

> The evidence obtained from the exercise highlighted information shortfalls in key areas such as housing, handling finances, the law and state benefits. At the same time there was over provision of information about health, sex and drugs. Young people were not impressed with lengthy typed text and preferred humour and graphics. They also preferred fewer items of information on the same topic, and were seeking more in the way of signposting, preferably from a 'one-stop' approach.
> (COIC/CSNU 2001: 6)

'Informing' in practice: Sasha

Sasha has called in to the centre to find out more about her idea of going to college to study information technology (IT). She tells you she has used the library at school and thinks she will be able to find what she needs. You show her where the college prospectuses are in the centre library, and give her a leaflet which summarises the IT courses available at the different campuses and gives information about how to contact the college, and about the application process. Sasha leaves a few minutes later, telling you that she now has the information she needs.

'Informing' in practice: Jan

Jan is waiting in the centre reception area for his friend who has an appointment with your colleague. He is looking at the information display, and picks up a leaflet for another helping agency and asks if he can take it. You ask if he would like to talk to someone but he tells you he just thought it looked interesting, and that he will call the number on the leaflet if he needs more help. You tell him that he can take the leaflet, and say that he can come back in future if he does want to talk to someone.

In these examples, the young people are provided with the information they want, but there is no discussion of it, as they do not feel it is necessary at this stage. Contact between the young people and the helper is minimal, but what is important is that the possibility remains for further discussion if the young person decides it would be of help.

Appropriate information is, therefore, important to young people. However, it is not enough on its own: 'Without an adequate base of information, none of the activities is possible, but a service which only seeks to provide information cannot, in any adequate way, meet the needs of its clients' (UDACE 1986: 25). Ways of helping clients to work with information will be considered in the section on skills and strategies in chapter 6.

Advising

Very often, when a young person has received information, they need to spend some time thinking about the implications of the information for their situation. As discussed previously, they may ask advice from a parent or carer, a teacher or a friend. This is frequently sufficient to enable them to move on. However, there may be reasons why a young person does not feel that they can talk to these other people, and they may seek advice from a professional helper. The advice gained from a professional helper should be qualitatively different from that gained from other people. For example, the helper can maintain an impartial approach in helping the young person to explore the information, as they do not have an agenda of their own. This may be in contrast to, for instance, a teacher who may be expected to promote options within the school. Also, the young person may be able to share factors that need to be taken into account that they would find difficult to talk to a parent or carer about. For example, in discussing personal relationships, the helper will be non-judgemental, and will not impose their own values on the young person. In this way, it may be easier for a young person to raise potentially challenging issues without being laughed at, which may happen with friends or peers (for example if a young person is considering non-traditional career choices, or is worried about their sexuality).

Advising in practice: Sasha

Sasha has returned to see you at the centre. She has looked on the college website, and has found a course called 'Foundation Course in Computing' but she is not sure whether it is the right one for her. Her form tutor has told her that she would be better staying at school for an AVCE course in Information and Communication Technology. She is also confused because her dad has told her that she won't get a job in IT, because she's a girl and she will be competing with boys who are better at IT. You decide to deal with her dad's comments first as she seems to be particularly concerned about his view. So (having taken a deep breath!), you ask Sasha if she agrees with what he said,

continued on next page

---

which she doesn't, and you ask her if she knows of any women in IT jobs, and she is able to identify several from the firm of IT consultants where she did her work experience. She decides that she will not be put off by her dad's remarks. You then suggest that together you go through the information she has about the two IT courses. The college course will give her the equivalent of four GCSEs at grades A–C, but she tells you she is expected to get six GCSEs at grades A–C this summer, so would not be any further forward. She likes the idea of going to college, but thinks that the AVCE may be more appropriate. Sasha is beginning to see how the information she found relates to her own situation.

Advising in practice: Jan

Jan calls back in to the centre to check that it will be OK if he calls the number on the leaflet he picked up. He thinks the agency may be able to help him, but wants to make sure that he won't need to give his name. Together you go through the information he has gleaned from the leaflet and you are able to confirm that the service is confidential, and that he can call any time. You are careful not to ask about the circumstances which mean that he feels this particular agency may be able to help him, but you make sure he knows he can come back to the centre in future if he wants to talk more.

One of the most important things about these examples is that the helper is careful to remain impartial and, unlike Sasha's dad or teacher, gives the young person the opportunity to think about the implications for them of the information they have and to begin to think about how they can take things forward. It is also important to allow young people adequate time and space to decide if they require more help – for some young people it will be enough to have considered the implications of the information for the next steps to become clear. For others, more help will be necessary, but it will only be beneficial if the young person has decided that this is what they want and need.

Counselling

The professional helper, in the context of this book, is not a counsellor; although the distinction may be less clear than we think in 'intensive' work (Westergaard 2003). There is a wealth of literature on therapeutic counselling that is readily available. The professional helper who is not a trained counsellor will often use the skills and strategies of counselling (Kidd 1996) to provide an impartial and non-judgemental arena in which a young person can explore issues for themselves. In this way helpers use the counselling skills derived from the work of Rogers (1951, 1961). At its simplest, this may mean providing a 'sounding board' so that the young person can try out ideas on someone who will not impose their own views. Key to this is the use of active listening, which will be dealt with further in the section on skills and strategies in chapter 6. When a helper listens and reflects back what has been said, a young person can 'hear' what they are saying. This provides an opportunity for the young person to identify any discrepancies in what they are saying, and to clarify their thoughts. The aim of the activity of counselling, within the helping relationship, is to give young people the time and space to work through issues for themselves, and can be a very useful way of helping them to identify their needs.

Let us take a step back to our first meeting with Sasha or Jan, and imagine an alternative scenario.

Counselling in practice: Sasha

Sasha has called into the centre, and asks about IT courses. You detect that she is hesitant about discussing this, but that she may want more than just the information. As you show her the prospectuses, you ask her about her idea of a career in IT. This gives her the opportunity to talk, and she tells you that she really enjoys IT at school, but is being put off taking the idea any further because her dad is against it, and has told her that she won't get a job in IT because she's a girl and she will be competing with boys who are better at IT. Sasha does not want to upset her dad, but she also knows that she is at least as good as any of the boys in her IT class, and has completed her work experience with a firm of IT consultants. Her dad was fine about this, as it was based in his office, and he thinks office work is OK for girls. She tells you that she has not been able to talk to anyone about it before, as her mum won't disagree with her dad, and her teacher just talks about going on to do further study at school rather than the college. You provide Sasha with time just to talk, and you are careful not to make any comments about what she is telling you – you remain non-judgemental.

Counselling in practice: Jan

Jan is looking at the information display, and picks up a leaflet for another helping agency, and asks if he can take it. You ask if he

continued on next page

would like to talk to someone, and he asks if you have time now, as he is very concerned about his older brother. As you are on duty, you are able to give him some time, and you take him to a private interview room. You ask him what he is worried about, and he tells you that his brother who is 19 is drinking heavily, and tends to get violent when he has been drinking. So far he has only damaged furniture, but Jan is worried that he may lash out at other members of the family. Quickly you recognise that this situation is beyond the boundary of your expertise, but you provide an opportunity for Jan to talk as it seems to help him. Eventually, he tells you that he knows his brother won't seek help, but that he would like some support. You explain that you are not an expert in this, but that there may be someone else who can help, and that it is likely that the agency he has identified will be a good starting point.

In these examples, the helper may well feel that there is little that they can actually do to help, but the fact that they can give the young person some space and time can in itself be supportive, and the young person may well find that they are clearer about the situation just from talking it through. In some situations the helper may be able to work on the issue, and in others they may need to refer the young person to someone with expertise in the area of concern. Two things are key here: remaining non-judgemental about what the young person is telling you, and being clear about the boundaries of your own expertise.

Assessing

For most people, 'assessment' means that they are being tested in some way, usually by someone else. This is certainly the case for young people, whose lives in school are circumscribed by various assessments at all stages: SATS (Standard Attainment Tests, the popular name for National Curriculum Tests), GCSEs, school tests, music exams, sports awards and so on. Many organisations working with young people will have formal assessment frameworks designed to assess the needs of the young people they serve. We are not dealing here with those formal assessment methods. In terms of our definition of 'helping activities', the responsibility is less with someone else, and much more with the young person. Assessing should be a shared activity, in which the young person and the helper work together to arrive at an understanding of the situation. Much of the information will come from the young person, and will include thoughts and feelings as much as facts. But, both the young person and the helper can also draw on information from a range of other sources, including family and friends, the school, other professionals, as well as from previous assessments, for example mock exam results or a Statement of Additional Educational Needs.

Assessing in practice: Sasha

Sasha is considering a course in IT, but is not entirely sure that it is right for her. You may want to encourage her to look at other options as well, but you don't want to impose your views on her. You suggest that she goes through the KUDOS computer package, which will give her an opportunity to think about her interests and likely qualifications, and will match these up with suggested career ideas. This may be enough, but you also offer her the chance to discuss with you the list of suggestions Sasha gets from KUDOS.

Assessing in practice: Jan

As Jan talks about his concerns in relation to his brother's drinking, you are already aware that you have reached the limit of your competence, and will need to find someone who is better placed to help him. You are weighing up in your mind the possibilities you know about, but you ask Jan to tell you what sort of help he thinks will be most beneficial. As you discuss this, Jan is beginning to identify for himself what he wants, and he discovers that he would prefer to talk to a person locally rather than call a helpline.

These examples show the different kinds of assessing that may take place with young people. In Sasha's case, a formal method of assessment is used, with the advantage that the helper is not tempted to impose their own ideas, but remains impartial. Very often, this type of assessment will raise questions for the young person, so they will want to discuss it further with a helper. For Jan, the process of assessing his situation and needs takes place as part of a discussion, where thoughts and feelings can all be taken into account, and he can decide what will be most helpful.

The aim of assessment within the helping relationship is to provide a full picture of the young person's situation, so that they have a sound basis for moving on. We will look at assessment again in chapter 4, when discussing the role of the youth support worker.

Enabling

Young people very often have a reasonably clear idea of *what* they hope to achieve, either in terms of their next steps or in relation to long term goals, even though they may require some help to clarify and share this with another person. The difficulty is very often in being clear about *how* to achieve their goals. The role of the helper is to support the young person in working out how to achieve their goals.

Coleman and Hendry (1999: 13), considering research into the lives of young people, suggest that 'the idea that the individual young person is an "active agent" in shaping or determining his or her own development has generally not been part of the thinking of researchers in this field'. As professional helpers, we are working with young people so that they can become active agents, and this is what we mean by 'enabling'. It may involve helping a young person to contact other agencies, such as colleges or training providers, and to follow this up with appropriate action to meet their needs. What is important is that the young person is able to take responsibility for the action because, as a result of the helping relationship, they understand what needs to be done to achieve their goals.

Enabling is often the most significant of the helping activities, as it means that the young person can begin to see how they can put their ideas into practice, and can begin to take responsibility for their actions.

Enabling in practice: Sasha

Having spent some time with Sasha, she is now clear about what she needs to do to move forward. In your discussion, she identifies several action steps that she needs to take. First she is going to find out more about the AVCE course at her school, as this seems to be the level of course she is looking for. You ask her who would be the best person to talk to about this, and she identifies her IT teacher. Second, as she still likes the idea of going to college, she wants to consider other courses there, including A levels. She has looked at the college website but wants to find out what it would be like to study there, so she suggests that she could talk to her cousin who is a student at the college. You tell her about the college Open Days, and she agrees that it would be useful to visit. She also decides that she would like to persuade her dad to go with her, so he can get a better idea of what she would be doing. Though she is still mainly interested in IT, she thinks it would be helpful to look at some of the other suggestions on the KUDOS list, so you check that she is clear about how to find out more – she knows about the Jobs4U website, and is happy to look things up on that.

You summarise, and between you write an action plan to remind her of the main things she is going to do.

Enabling in practice: Jan

Jan knows he wants to talk to someone about his brother's drinking and the impact this is having on the family. He understands that you are not able to help him further and he would like to talk to someone who knows about this kind of issue. You know of two local agencies that may be able to help, so you explain what each one does and Jan decides which sounds most likely to be of help.

The young person operating as an 'active agent' who feels in control of their next steps, is the key to effective enabling.

Advocating

Young people are often not confident to speak up for themselves, particularly when they need to deal with adults. It may be part of the role of the professional helper to act as an advocate on behalf of a young person, or, indeed, on behalf of a group of young people. In using the term 'advocate', we need to be aware that we are not using it in the legal sense of the word, as a barrister would understand the term. Rather, we are acting as a supporter for young people, in giving them an opportunity to get their point of view across, and, if they are not able to speak for themselves, to do this for them. It is important that, as professional helpers, we do this in a professional way. Ideally, this involves a significant amount of preparation, in helping the young person to be clear about what they do want to say, and in clarifying how far they want us to act on their behalf. Of course, it is not always possible to spend time in preparation before advocating: the need for the activity often arises because of a crisis.

Bateman (1995) identifies two main types of problem, which necessitate advocating on behalf of a young person. First, 'bounded problems' are those in which the situation can be resolved fairly quickly, because the solution to the problem is clearly identified and can be worked towards independently of other issues. Second, 'unbounded problems': these are less clear as factors which will have an impact on a solution are more complex, so the implications are greater, but more uncertain. Working as an advocate for a young person is less complex for bounded problems, and may involve only one session. Unbounded problems are likely to need more ongoing work, and often the first stage is to help the young person to identify priorities as not everything can be resolved immediately. Young people who require more intensive support are likely to need help with unbounded problems.

Bateman (1995) also suggests six principles that should underpin advocacy. He uses the term 'Principled Advocacy', and it is this approach which we can apply to professional helpers. The six principles, adapted slightly to fit the context of work with young people, are:

- Act in the young person's best interests.
- Act in accordance with the young person's wishes and instructions.
- Keep the young person properly informed.
- Carry out instructions with diligence and competence.
- Act impartially and offer frank, independent advice.
- Maintain confidentiality.

It is essential to keep these principles in mind when advocating on a young person's behalf. They can also act as a reminder that advocacy is not something which should be undertaken lightly, especially in relation to unbounded problems.

Advocating in practice: Sasha

Sasha is generally confident in speaking and doing things for herself, but it is possible to envisage situations where she may feel the need for more support. If she is feeling pressured by the school to stay on after GCSEs, she may find it helpful for you to speak to her form tutor or head of year. This can help to set the scene and to explain what she wants to discuss with them so that she doesn't get flustered when she sees them. A slightly more difficult situation could arise if Sasha felt that she needed support in talking to her dad about her ideas about a career in IT, and his attitude to this. You will need to be very clear about what she wants you to say to him on her behalf, and to make sure he understands that this is what you are doing. However, it may well help to have a dispassionate outsider (you) to speak for Sasha, and it may help to overcome some of the difficulties she perceives.

Advocating in practice: Jan

This may well be a significant part of the help you provide to Jan. He may not feel confident enough to contact agencies, and may be concerned that he will be unable to express clearly what he wants and needs from them. This can be very daunting for anyone. So, you will work with him to decide what he wants you to say on his behalf, and to formulate any questions he may need to have answered. You will then contact the agency on his behalf, ideally while Jan is still with you – there are several advantages in this: Jan will know that you are saying what he wants said, he will be able to answer any subsequent questions from the agency, he will feel that he has made contact with people at the agency and he may feel enabled to speak to them himself, once the scene has been set. Your intervention here will mean that it will be possible for Jan to undertake future contact with the agency himself.

In these examples, the helper takes time to ensure that they are clear about what the young person wants to say, and does not add anything without checking first with the young person. In addition, the fact that the helper is 'outside' the situation can help the young person's voice to be heard, without the emotional layers which are likely in sensitive situations and which may mask the message they want to express.

Ideally, young people should be able to speak for themselves, and, as professional helpers, we will be encouraging them to do so. On occasions when they are not able to speak for themselves, we may need to advocate on their behalf. Working alongside a young person, and ensuring they have the opportunity to take an active part in the process, will deter us from assuming a powerful position that takes away their independence – however 'fledgling' this independence may be. Our role is to help young people move on, so we would hope to build their confidence and their ability to speak independently, to enable them to advocate on their own behalf in the future.

Feeding back

As professional helpers, we are working with young people who are of an age when they are likely to be unsure about their identity. Coleman and Hendry (1999: 27) suggest that 'the development of the individual's identity requires not only the notion of being separate and different from others, but also a sense of self-consistency and a firm knowledge of how one appears to the rest of the world'. Uncertainty about identity can often lead young people to try out lots of different 'selves' in their attempt to establish themselves as separate, or different, from their parents and other adults. Consequently, their behaviour or appearance may, at times, appear to the adults in their lives as challenging or inappropriate. It is the role of the professional helper to enable young people to see for themselves how they appear to the rest of the world, so that they can make choices about any changes they may need to make, either in behaviour or appearance, in order to achieve their goals. Coleman and Hendry (1999: 27) also state that, 'It is unfortunate that many adults – even those in teaching and similar professions – retain only a vague awareness of the psychological impact of the physical changes associated with puberty'. It is, perhaps, understandable that many people will wish to forget what may have been an uncomfortable stage in their lives. However, it is invaluable for those involved in helping young people to retain some understanding of this, so that we can both relate to young people's feelings and help them to see themselves as others do. Again, it is important to be non-judgemental, and to avoid imposing our own values on young people, so that they can make their own choices.

Feeding back in practice: Sasha

Sasha is angry at her dad's attitude to her interest in IT, and tells you that they have had several rows about it, neither of them being prepared to back down. You can understand her point of view, but you ask her if she knows why her dad thinks in this way. She is not sure and has not asked him, but thinks it may be because he worked in an engineering firm where there was a girl apprentice who was given a hard time by the 'lads', and also by the other girls who worked in the offices. She sees that he may be trying to protect her from a similar experience. You also ask her how she responds to him, and she tells you she usually loses her temper and storms out. She says that she would like to be able to talk to him properly, but needs to control her temper, so you discuss how she could do this. We have seen how advocating on Sasha's behalf could be one way of getting over this, but if Sasha can work through it herself, so she can talk to her dad, she will be beginning to take responsibility for herself.

Feeding back in practice: Jan

At the moment, Jan is confused and unhappy about the impact of his brother's drinking on the family. As he is the one who intervenes when his brother comes home drunk and violent, he has received most of the unpleasantness himself. He has begun to feel that he is in some way to blame, and this is not helped by his mum who tells him to leave his brother alone, as Jan is 'making things worse'. You recognise that this is a fairly common reaction, but that you need to help Jan to understand that it is not his fault. You ask him to tell you what happens, and he begins to see that he is feeling guilty because he is the one caught 'in the middle'. You and Jan agree that when you refer him to an agency who can help, you will mention that this is something he wants to work through.

In these examples, the problem is not solved, but the young person has recognised that there is something which needs to be changed or worked on. More importantly, they have some ideas about what they can do to move forward.

Networking

The *Chambers Dictionary* (1988) defines a network as 'any structure in the form of a net . . . a system of units, e.g. groups of people constituting a widely spread organisation and having a common purpose. A group of people who share information, swap contacts etc.' A network, then, is a linking of people who have some purpose in common, and a shared reason to stay in contact with one another. In the case of professional helpers working with young people, the networks they are involved in would constitute other individuals and agencies who also work with young people, and who have complementary skills and expertise. Networks can be informal; for example the contacts that an individual helper has made in the course of their work, or formal; where a group is set up with a particular remit and an organisational structure. The advantage of informal networks is that they can be very flexible and responsive, and work on the basis of mutual help. The disadvantage is that they may not always contain an appropriate contact, and the information is often lost when the individual helper leaves or moves on. Formal networks, which often take the form of directories of other agencies, work best at organisational level. A shared directory may ensure that information is not lost; but is less helpful if the needs of the young person fall outside its remit. In the latter case, personal contact can prove more useful.

Exercise in networking

It is useful for helpers working with young people to consider the quality of the networking they do, as this can ensure appropriate and effective referrals. You can follow the steps below to check your own relationships with key people and organisations in your network:

- List as many actual network contacts which you use in your work with young people.
- Rate these on a scale of 1–5 in importance to your work. 1 is low, 5 is high importance.
- Now rate them in terms of the quality of the networking relationship. A = good, B = OK, C = needs attention.
- In the centre of a piece of paper draw a circle to represent you. From this circle, draw a line to represent each contact and name it. Put those which rate highest in importance closest to you, and the less important farther away.
- Now mark each contact with the letter which indicates the quality of the relationship.

You now have a 'map' of your network contacts and can begin to address the questions which can help to improve your networking: Are there any of high importance where the relationship needs work? Why are these contacts more difficult? What can be done about this?

Networking is a key activity for helpers working with young people, and the networks can provide an invaluable source of support. It must be stressed, however, that networking is not just about getting to know as many people as possible. Your network must be able to provide specific contacts who can help you in meeting the needs of the young people you work with.

Networking in practice: Sasha

In working with Sasha you are drawing on a wide range of networking contacts to ensure that the help you give her is as effective as possible. You will draw on your knowledge of the local college, the courses they offer, and the most useful people to contact. You will also link into your networks within the school, to ensure that Sasha gets the support she needs. If you are not familiar with the school yourself, you will need to talk to colleagues who are. This may seem so obvious that you do not recognise it as networking, but it is making sure that you use your contacts as effectively as possible to support Sasha.

Networking in practice: Jan

Jan's specific need means that you may need to contact other agencies who can help him. You may already be aware of these, so will have some knowledge of what they can offer. If you are not familiar with local organisations which can help, you will need to find out what is available. This may be achieved by asking colleagues, but you may also have access to a local directory of such agencies, which can give you information about the help they offer: for example, who they are able to help, and if there are any restrictions on this, such as age limits. In many cases we prefer the more personal approach, as we can perhaps find out more directly about the outcomes they have achieved for other young people. This may well reassure Jan, but we may have to recognise that this personal approach will not always be possible.

Referring

One of the things a professional helper must be particularly aware of is the limit of their own competence and expertise. This may sound like an admission of inability to do the job, but it is, in essence, the opposite. Because many of the young people we work with have very complicated lives, and consequently very complex needs, it is not possible for one person to meet all the needs of all young people. We will each have our own areas of knowledge and expertise, which make us the right person to help young people with issues or problems related to those areas. These areas of knowledge and expertise also mean that we may be the wrong person to help with issues and problems which fall outside of them. In these circumstances, we need to refer a young person on to someone better placed to offer the appropriate help. This awareness of the limits of our expertise leads to 'ethical watchfulness' (Reid 2002) and is essential for effective helping to take place within an ethical framework.

For example, my areas of knowledge and expertise are career guidance and helping students in college as their tutor. If I am working with a young person who is considering a career choice, or looking at the possibility of going to university, I am able to help that young person because their needs fall within my areas of knowledge and expertise. If, in the course of a discussion, the young person tells me that they have had to leave home, and have been sleeping on a friend's floor for a week, I am able to offer basic help to clarify the problem, but cannot deal with it myself. I would need to refer the young person on to someone who could offer the specialist help they need. I would have reached the limit of my competence, recognised this, and continued to help the young person by finding someone else who can deal with those aspects that are outside of the boundaries of my expertise.

This is referral, and for referrals to be effective, you need to:

- Make sure the young person knows exactly who you are referring them to, and why.
- Make sure the young person knows what information will be shared, and that they give their informed consent to this.
- Make sure the young person understands how the referral will benefit them.
- Make sure the young person does not feel you are just passing them on elsewhere.
- Make sure you take time to ensure they know they can come back to you if necessary.
- Make sure they know exactly what will happen.
- Make sure the young person is involved in the referral process, for example:

    1 Complete any paperwork, e.g. referral form, with them, so they know what is written.
    2 Contact the other organisation or individual while they are there, and if possible let the young person speak to someone.
    3 Ensure the young person has all the relevant contact information.
    4 Indicate if it is possible for you to go with them if they wish: this can be very supportive.

- Make sure you follow up the referral to see how they got on.

The referral should always be in the best interest of the young person. It may not require referring them to an external organisation, but could be an internal referral to a colleague with a different area of knowledge and expertise. As suggested earlier, many referrals rely on the personal contacts and networks of the individual helper, so their effectiveness is dependent on the quality of those contacts. Confidentiality (and its limits) needs to be discussed in any interaction, but will need to be reviewed before agreeing a referral (Daniels and Jenkins 2000; Brown 2003). Similarly, you will need to review the 'rules' or codes of practice for recording information within your organisation, and the protocols for sharing that information between the agencies involved.

Referring in practice: Sasha

If you see Sasha in the centre when you are on duty, you may feel that you can deal with her immediate need to find out about IT courses at college, but that your expertise is not in career guidance. You may find that she needs to talk to a colleague who has this expertise – you are aware that you may even do harm by getting into this, if she does not consider all the implications – so you will make an appointment for Sasha to come back to see a career guidance practitioner. This is an internal referral.

Referring in practice: Jan

As you talk to Jan, it has become increasingly clear that he is going to need much more specialised help and support than you can provide. Jan also understands this, and, after you have discussed issues around confidentiality and information sharing, he is happy to go to see someone else who will be able to help him. You have drawn on your network of contacts, to agree an agency that may well be able to help, and Jan is ready to be referred to them. You have spoken to them already (advocating) to put across Jan's situation (without naming him) and to check that they will be able to help. You are now in a position to make a formal referral, and you check with the agency what they need from you to ensure that this can happen – it may be that the phone call is sufficient and you can make the appointment for Jan, but it is likely that there will be a form to complete. You do this with Jan, so that he knows what has been written. You also agree that you will contact him later to see how things are going and to check that the referral has been useful for Jan. You make sure that he knows he can come back in future if things do not work out. With a referral to an external organisation, you need to ensure that there is an 'open door' so the young person can return.

Referring a young person to other agencies or colleagues is not an admission of incompetence, but a professional judgement based on a recognition that you have reached the limit of your competence. Referral must always be in the best interest of the young person – they need to understand and agree the need for the referral.

Of course, there are times when it feels like we are 'the end of the line' with nowhere else to refer the young person on to. When this happens the situation needs to be brought to the attention of senior managers in an organisation, who will need to lobby for action from the relevant agencies or funding bodies. Perhaps 'lobbying' should be another activity of helping!

Summary

In this chapter we have explored a range of activities that help to define the working context for the youth support worker. It must be stressed that not all the helping activities will be appropriate for meeting the needs of a young person. The skill of the professional helper lies in making some decisions about which activities to use and when. The helping activities are all closely related, and while you are unlikely to need to use all of them in helping any individual young person, we have seen from the examples how they can work together, and how one can lead to the next. The helping activities should be seen as a menu of possibilities, not a checklist to be followed.

In conclusion, the helping relationship encompasses a number of activities which can be used by the professional helper in working with a young person to meet their needs. The helping activities are separate, yet interrelated, so that they can be used in combination to help a young person to work towards positive outcomes. What we mean by positive outcomes is discussed further in chapter 5; before that the next chapter considers the context for the helping activities described above.

4   The helping context

Introduction

The central aim of this book is to help practitioners structure their helping relationships with young people. As noted earlier, professional helping can be delivered through a wide range of interventions, not just via one-to-one interviews, which may be the most common, but are not the only form of help available to young people. Helping activities, considered in the previous chapter, contribute to the helping process and can involve a variety of methods. Methods could be described as interventions, and this chapter considers helping interventions alongside the role of the youth support worker/professional helper in the helping context. As in previous chapters, examples and exercises are included to relate the concepts discussed to practice.

A helping intervention

Definition:

> A helping intervention is any event or experience which affects or contributes towards the young person's feelings, knowledge and thinking about issues, plans, ideas or decisions that they intend to act upon.

The event or experience may be positive or negative or even neutral, and may not even be an intentional contribution to the young person's progress through the helping process. For example, the most obvious helping event is the one-to-one meeting between the young person and the youth support worker. This meeting is a planned contribution towards the helping process. It is an identifiable intervention in that the practitioner intervenes in a positive sense, between the young person and their experience, ideas and feelings about a given situation or plan.

The one-to one meeting

Dev has called in to the centre to see his youth support worker. He has been looking for work since he left college, but he has had no luck. He has found the situation quite depressing and finds it difficult to motivate himself to get up in the morning – he was 15 minutes late for his 2.30 pm appointment. His helper discovers that he has missed the last two job interviews because they were in the morning. Between them, Dev and his helper identify some strategies to address this issue: his next few appointments will be arranged at progressively earlier times, to encourage a gradual return to getting up in the morning; he will make sure he sets the alarm on his mobile phone, and agrees to text his helper to let them know that he is awake; his helper will call Dev's mobile in plenty of time before his next job interview to make sure that he doesn't miss it. Dev leaves feeling more positive, and confident that he will be able to do what has been agreed.

Another fairly obvious intervention is where a young person participates in a group activity with others in a similar situation or with similar needs. The group session is an intervention offered by the helping agency or practitioner as a means of helping the young person to achieve a positive outcome.

The group session

Sara is a teenage parent who missed taking her GCSEs because of the birth of her daughter. She is living in a rented flat and feels very isolated, because it is a long way from her family and friends. She is no longer with her baby's father. Her youth support worker has suggested she comes to the centre to join a newly formed group of teenage parents, with the aim of sharing experiences and providing some support to one another.

Sara attends the session and meets up with four other young women who are in a similar situation. She finds that one of them lives in her own block of flats. They discuss their experiences, find a lot in common, and have a good laugh. They agree that they would like to meet regularly, and discover that their helper can arrange some activities related to bringing up their children. They also exchange mobile phone numbers so they can keep in touch. Sara leaves feeling less isolated already, and is looking forward to the next session.

In contrast to those planned interventions, unintentional interventions are those where an event or experience occurs that has no direct link to formal helping, whether from the professional or friends. An unintended intervention is where something happens which affects the young person's ideas or feelings about their situation or plans. For instance, a young person may need help with making a decision (which they may or may not have sought formal help with). The young person happens to be chatting to someone about their issue, ideas, feelings or plans, just because that person is there; is willing to listen; or has experience that is relevant.

An unintentional intervention

Hanna is intending to go on to do A-levels at school, as she will be with many of her friends and she will know the teachers. At a family party she meets up with her cousin who is talking about her experience at college. Hanna does not take part in the conversation, but listens to everything and begins to get a picture of college as somewhere exciting and different from school, rather than somewhere daunting and unfriendly. She starts to think that she may find out more about the college and the courses on offer.

It may be that a young person responds to something someone says just because it is a person they trust. This can happen at a friend's house, at a party, on a bus or when just 'hanging out' somewhere.

A chance comment

Davy is hanging around with a group of mates in the local park. One of his friends mentions that the local youth forum is trying to persuade the council to build a five-a-side all weather football pitch on some derelict ground nearby. Davy is a dedicated footballer, and he thinks this sounds like a good idea. He finds out when the next forum meeting is, goes along and offers to help with fund raising for the project. He also gets involved in other activities with the forum, becomes one of the leaders in the group and eventually becomes Chair. When he applies to university, his involvement in the youth forum is a positive factor in his being offered a place.

So, any ideas, information or feelings that result from an experience or an event that affect the individual's thinking about their own situation, and which contribute to their subsequent decisions, turn the experience or event into an intervention in the helping process – whether this was an intended outcome or not.

As practitioners, we need to take unintentional interventions and informal helping into account, as sometimes these can be more influential for a young person than expert and formal interventions. As such, it is important to be aware of the social context of the young person on the receiving end of professional helping. In other words their lives outside of the helping relationship will impact on any intervention we take. Any interventions are related to context and can inform and enhance the helping process for the young person. That context may include interventions organised by the helping agency in which you work, or a related agency that is part of the helping network for work with young people.

A variety of interventions to meet individual needs

Helping agencies and youth support workers need to think carefully about the methods that they use to deliver their services to young people, in order to cater for individual preferences and learning styles (Honey and Mumford 1992). By learning styles we mean the individual's preferred way of acquiring knowledge and skills or dealing with information and new ideas. Thus, helping agencies and practitioners should be able to provide a range of ways in which they offer help to young people. These should include both structured and unstructured events and experiences. For example, an information browsing service is an unstructured method of providing support, which a young person may be able to use on their own. A structured helping intervention might include the opportunity to use an IT package, with or without the assistance of a helper. A young person who requires minimal support may only need the address and telephone number of a referral agency; others will need the practitioner to accompany them and may require the helper to speak on their behalf.

Additional support might include some of the following, depending on the resources available and the context (some of these were discussed in the previous chapter under helping activities):

- follow-up of young people – few will be sorted in one session;
- referral to other agencies, with the young person's consent;
- working with parents and care-givers or community representatives;
- advocacy;
- a range of structured and unstructured group activities – this may include organising events in outreach locations;
- access to resources, facilities and a range of technologies;

- testing and assessment;
- providing and sending information to young people;
- arranging visits to other agencies, institutions, educational establishments, employers, sources of information and so on.

Contextual awareness

Of course, what we do and how we do it will depend on key factors pertinent to the young person we are working with – to that end we need to be flexible in our approach and the use of any model. There are several approaches within counselling that may be particularly relevant for working with young people. Space precludes a discussion of these approaches here, but the reference list will indicate further reading.

When considering the impact of the social context on any young person, a consideration of multiculturalism from the counselling literature will be relevant. Whilst multiculturalism is a well-established concept within counselling and psychotherapy, its principles are less likely to be located within the intervention models used for professional helping. Training does pay attention to equal opportunities, but often this remains politically neutral and does not consider the multi-layered subjects of social justice and multiculturalism. Both concepts are frequently viewed as a concern with ethnicity rather than with a range of variables linked to social context. The term multiculturalism in the context of helping is, then, wider than ethnicity and relates to any potential barrier to benefit from 'goods and services'.

The approach used in this book is derived from the humanistic work of Rogers (1951, 1961) and Egan (2002). However, these approaches have been criticised as dependent on a 'world view' that is white, 'Western', Anglo-Saxon and Protestant (WASP). What critics suggest is that adaptations to a three-stage helping model, or in some cases an entirely different model, are required to cater for the needs of young people whose 'worldviews' are different from each other and different from that of the practitioner. For example, for some young people a Rogerian approach, which assumes that the individual can motivate change, is in direct contrast to their lived experience where it is the family or the community that makes decisions about future plans. As practitioners, and to go beyond empathy, we should be aware of our own cultural values and consider how they influence the approaches we take to working with young people. Even when from the same cultural group, the values of the young person and the practitioner may be very different.

Again this is a topic that cannot be given adequate coverage here, but readers may like to research this further from the counselling and guidance literature (Sue *et al.* 1996; Fouad and Bingam 1995; Bimrose 1996; Fielding 1999; Reid 2005). Finding out about other approaches and integrating these into our practice helps us to develop 'knowledgeable practice' (Edwards

1998), a step up from practical knowledge gained from the use of one helping model. That said, what we use in practice will be based on our assessment of 'what works', with particular young people in particular
circumstances. Our experience suggests that the three-stage model of helping
(the Single Interaction Model), based on Egan, is a good place to start.

Role of the youth support worker

The role of the youth support worker (YSW) is complex, and involves co-
ordinating work with many other individuals and agencies, as well as ensuring that the needs of the young person are kept at the centre of any work.
The role is presented in diagrammatic form (figure 4.1) to give an overview
of the many aspects involved, and to show the relationships between the
different areas. The youth support worker is shown as central, because of
the co-ordinating role they undertake, but it must be remembered that the
purpose of the work is meeting the needs of the young person, albeit that
we have placed the youth support worker in the centre of the diagram.
The process that can frame different aspects of the role (SIM) is clarified in
chapter 7. The role falls into two main parts: the direct work with the
young person, and the brokerage work with other agencies and individuals.
We will consider each of these in turn with reference to figure 4.1.

Direct work

The first aspect of direct work with a young person is **assessment**. (We looked
at assessment in the previous chapter and intimated there how separate
activities need to be integrated into the whole process.) This is the point at
which the referral of a young person to the youth support worker is
accepted. It is important that the helper, sometimes in consultation with
their line manager, is clear that the referral is appropriate and that they
are the 'best' person to undertake the work. In order to ensure that this is
the case, the helper will need to gather information from the referrer, but
may also need to discuss needs directly with the young person – they are
often the best source of information about their own situation. It is unlikely
that a full and formal assessment method (one example would be the
Connexions' Assessment, Planning, Implementation and Review tool –
APIR) will be completed in its entirety at this stage. However, considering
the information gathered in relation to factors in an assessment tool can
give a good indication of the appropriateness, or not, of the referral. If it
is judged that the referral is appropriate, figure 2.4 (page 21) provides the
practitioner with a means to identify the likely level of the young person's
needs. At this point, referral to more specialist help may be necessary if the
young person has a specific and complex need that is outside your expertise.

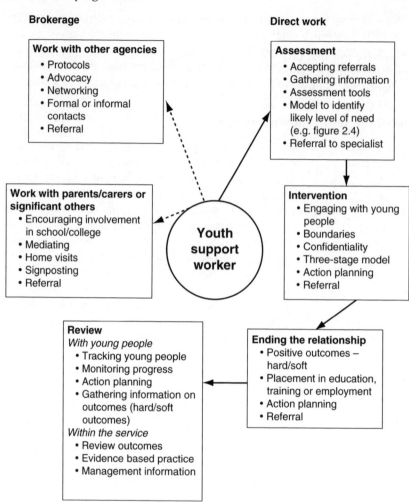

Figure 4.1 The role of the youth support worker.

An initial contact: Ben

You have just met Ben. He has come along with his friend who has an appointment with you.

Ben is 16, and in Year 11. He is supposed to be taking his mock GCSEs next week, but tells you that he can't be bothered to go in to school for them as it will be a waste of time. Instead, he will spend the time at the local skate park with his mates, many of whom have already left school. He is confident, articulate and communicative when talking to you. He was interested in what his friend had told him about the meetings with you, so he had come along to see whether you would be able to help him. He tells you that he has nowhere to live at the moment, as he left home after a row with his mum's boyfriend. He has been staying at his friend's house. He talks quite openly about the fact that, within the group he spends time with, there is quite a lot of drinking and some use of cannabis, and that he has, on occasion, joined in.

He won't discuss school, exams or his future.

What is your immediate response to what Ben has told you? This may well depend on your role, but consider the following possibilities:

- You are worried when he mentions that he has nowhere to stay as you are not an expert on housing issues, and you know that you are not able to help with drink and drug problems. You suggest that Ben may like to talk to a colleague of yours.
- You offer to call the local young people's housing trust to make an appointment for Ben.
- You engage Ben in conversation in the hope that he will tell you a bit more about his situation, so you can act accordingly.

All of these responses could prove helpful, and you will want to do what you both agree is most helpful for the immediate situation. Whatever decision you take it will be helpful to Ben in the long run if you don't rush things. While you have the chance to talk to him you may gain greater insight in order to make an informed decision about what you should do now and what you could do next time.

Earlier we discussed the development of the helping relationship with the young person when describing the range of interventions. In figure 4.1, **intervention** involves engaging with the young person, and it needs to be recognised that although the relationship between the young person and the helper is voluntary, it may still take some time for the young person to feel comfortable with the relationship; especially where trust may need to be worked on due to the young person's previous experiences. The helper needs to be clear about the boundaries of the relationship – what their role is, what they can and cannot help with, when they are available to the young person, and so on – and should ensure that the young person is also clear about this. In the same way, the helper needs to make sure that the young person understands the limits of confidentiality in the relationship: what can remain confidential, and what the helper would need to take action on or share with other people.

Working with young people who may be engaged in illegal activity, or those who may indicate that they are being abused or are abusing others, places the practitioner in a difficult situation. Practitioners must be clear about the relevant codes of practice for their organisation and work within these. However, we can be placed in situations that are not 'clear cut', where making a decision about what we do, or do not, take action over presents us with an ethical dilemma, particularly when we are working within a young person-focused approach (Daniels and Jenkins 2000; Mulvey 2002). In this situation, always seek advice from a line manager as soon as is possible and discuss any uncertainties within supervision. And if you do not have a system of support and supervision within your organisation, the experience will provide a good rationale to request that a system is initiated (Reid and Westergaard 2006).

Returning to our diagram (figure 4.1), the Single Interaction Model provides a framework for each intervention, and can be used to provide structure even when several meetings are required to meet the young person's needs. Key to this development is action planning, so that at the end of each meeting the young person and the helper are clear about what needs to be done before the next meeting. Action planning ensures that the helping relationship remains purposeful, and that the young person is moving forward towards achieving their goals, albeit by small steps. As the relationship develops it may become apparent that the youth support worker cannot help the young person further, and referral to another professional or agency may be needed.

Now consider the following

In the course of a discussion with Ben, he tells you that he usually gets on well with his mum's boyfriend, and sometimes goes fishing with him, and apart from fishing, they talk about sport. Ben is very keen on his skateboarding, and would really like to do this professionally. He is not able to concentrate on his exams because he is upset, but would really like to be able to do his GCSEs so he can go to college to do a GNVQ in leisure and tourism. The mates he sees at the skate park are mostly at college. He stayed at a mate's house last night, but his mate's mum says he must phone his own mum before she'll let him stay again. Ben thinks he'll probably be able to go home if the row has 'blown over'.

As the helper, what would your response be now? You will probably feel that with only a little help from you, Ben will be able to sort things out, and you can support him to do this.

The situation may not always be as straightforward as this, and we may need to spend more time making sure we understand the key issues in the young person's life; before we make any decisions about how far to engage with that young person.

An alternative scenario

How would you respond in this situation?

In the course of a discussion with Ben, he tells you that he had finally left home after a huge row with his mum's boyfriend, Dave. Ben does not get on with him at all, and has been on the receiving end of the man's violent temper, usually after Dave has been drinking. Ben shows you bruises on his arms. The cause of the final row was that Ben had been caught, by Dave, with some of his mates, who were smoking cannabis. Ben had defended this by saying that the behaviour was no worse than Dave's drinking. Dave lost his temper, grabbed Ben by the arm and hit him several times. Ben has now been sleeping on the floor at his mate's squat for four nights. His friends are supportive in that they tell him not to worry, but they don't have any practical ideas. Ben is concerned for his younger brother in case Dave 'takes it out on him', and for his mum, who doesn't know where he is.

continued on next page

You will soon realize that this situation will be more difficult to resolve, and may take some time, as well as involving other people: probably Ben's mum, and possibly other agencies. At this point you may feel that it is appropriate to refer Ben to someone who is able to offer specialist help. On the other hand, this may well be within your role, so you want to work with Ben to identify the main priorities at the moment, and to begin to put support in place. Your 'intervention' is likely to be quite prolonged.

Thinking about what we have covered so far in this chapter, are there any other issues here that need thinking about? If there are, how are you going to decide what to do next?

In a helping relationship where the young person is enabled to move forward to achieve their goals, there will come a point when they no longer need the help of the youth support worker. It is important that the helper recognises that the young person is less dependent, and can move forward independently: so **ending the relationship** is appropriate. This can be quite difficult for both the helper and the young person, but it is one of the things that characterizes professional helping relationships, in contrast to our informal or social relationships. In ending the relationship, the helper and the young person will be able to identify positive outcomes. These outcomes may be 'hard', such as placement in education, training or employment, or 'soft' (Dewson *et al.* 2000): for example the young person's self-confidence is now high enough that they are able to move forward without their helper. It is important that these outcomes are recognised, and celebrated, by both the young person and the helper, and action planning at this stage will ensure that momentum is not lost. Ending the relationship may happen as a result of referral to another practitioner or agency, but in most cases the youth support worker will want to make sure that the young person knows that they can return if they need help in the future.

Review

It is necessary to follow up young people for a number of reasons, so **review** (figure 4.1) is a key aspect of the role and has two main dimensions. Review with young people will involve tracking and monitoring their progress towards achieving their goals, and may include some additional action planning, particularly if the young person has come up against an unexpected barrier. Gathering information on outcomes will enable the helper to identify any unmet needs, and may involve referral to another practitioner or agency, but will also enable the helper to close cases. This links to review within the service, in that the youth support worker will be able to identify patterns in outcomes, and contribute to evidence based practice through sharing and dissemination of good practice. Equally important is the provision of management information, which informs planning and development within the service, including caseload allocation.

Brokerage

The brokerage aspect of the role (figure 4.1) is very significant in enabling the youth support worker to meet the needs of the young person. It is essential that the helper remembers that any work with other people or agencies should be focused on the young person's needs. **Work with parents/carers or significant others** may be difficult, but may also have a significant impact on the ability of the young person to move forward. At its most straightforward, this may involve encouraging involvement in school or college. More complex situations may involve the helper in mediating in family discussions, perhaps through home visits. The helper may feel that additional help beyond their remit might be needed, and they could be involved in 'signposting' to appropriate services, or in referral to specialist agencies, for example to family mediation services. Think about the alternative scenario for Ben, and consider how you could help him to contact his Mum, or what additional help may be needed. For some young people, the most important people in their lives may not be family members, but could be their partner or friends, and the youth support worker may find it helpful to engage with these 'significant others' as they can also offer support to the young person.

Work with other agencies is key in ensuring that the helper is able to offer the most appropriate help to a young person, and is dependent on local protocols (for example information sharing) being in place. The youth support worker may need to work with other agencies in an advocacy role, where the young person is not able to speak for themselves. The helper may draw on both formal and informal contacts, to meet the needs of the young person most appropriately. Referral to other agencies is one aspect of this, and the helper needs to be in contact with a wide range of other agencies so that each young person's needs can be met effectively. In Ben's case, this could involve a referral to a family mediation service, or maybe to the local housing department.

The direct work with young people and the brokerage aspects of the role are interdependent, and, where both are in place, will ensure that young people are enabled to move forward towards achieving their goals, within a purposeful helping relationship.

Summary

In this chapter we have considered helping interventions, the helping context and the role of the youth support worker, reflecting on the ethical nature of the work. The discussion has highlighted how diverse, complex, challenging and potentially rewarding the role of the youth support worker can be. If new to the work it probably sounds rather daunting! Perhaps it is worth stating that you will not be working alone. Even if your work context is relatively isolated, you will have a line manager and, as suggested earlier, hopefully access to structured support and supervision. It has been emphasised that when considering the context and organisational structure, the needs of the young person must remain central. This young person-focused approach is the subject of the following chapter.

5   The young person-focused approach

Introduction

Thus far in the book we have considered definitions, purpose, context, the helping process, helping activities and the role of the professional helper. Before moving on to look at helping skills, strategies and the three-stage Single Interaction Model later in the book, this chapter will discuss the wider aspects of a collaborative helping approach. We will consider the theoretical foundations of the young person-centred approach and identify the possible limitations of approaches derived from humanistic counselling. The chapter will also refer to the need to evaluate practice through identifying the positive outcomes of helping interventions, and will end with a discussion of aspects that contribute to effective helping.

The young person-focused approach

The client-centred, or what was later called the person-centred, approach is associated mainly with the work of Carl Rogers (1951, 1961). Rogers wrote extensively about person-centred therapy over a period of years and his best known work is probably *On Becoming a Person*, which was first published in 1961. Although Rogers' ideas were developed for psychotherapy, the principles of a person-centred approach have found validity and application in counselling and helping work that is non-therapeutic. Rogers also discussed how a person-centred approach could be applied to group and teaching situations. Whilst person-centred therapy remains a distinct approach, counsellors and workers in a wide range of professional helping settings have adopted many of the ideas put forward by Rogers.

The person-centred model is built on core principles relating to both the counsellor and the person being helped. In order to avoid clumsiness we will use the term 'client' here, although we are mindful that the person-centred approach of Rogers developed as a reaction to the labelling implications of that word. First of all, the person-centred model assumes that the client is an equal in the counsellor–client relationship. Also, it assumes that the client can take responsibility for their own behaviour and decisions, and in their own way, rather than pleasing the counsellor. In other words, the essence of the relationship is to enable and empower the client to take control of their own life.

In addition to the equality and responsibility ascribed to the client, Rogers postulated that the attitudes of the counsellor were of crucial importance. He identified three attitudinal qualities that he claimed were essential to the promotion of the 'actualising' or empowering process for the client. These are genuineness, respect and empathy. Genuineness, in that the counsellor is open and honest with the client about their attitudes and feelings towards the client: that is, being real or congruent within the relationship. Respect, in that the counsellor is able to demonstrate 'unconditional positive regard' for the client; in other words, the counsellor will accept the client's ideas and behaviour in a non-judgemental way. Empathy, in that the counsellor attempts to understand the client and the client's world as if they were that person – as far as that is possible.

To summarise, the key qualities of a client or person-centred approach are, for the client:

- the experience of equality within the counselling relationship;
- the recognition of their responsibility and control over their own lives.

And, from the counsellor:

- attitudinal qualities of genuineness, respect and empathy.

The young person-focused approach we outline in this book is derived from the work of Rogers but also takes into account criticisms of a humanistic approach.

Criticisms of the humanistic approach: the quest for goal- and action-orientated behaviour

The approach advocated in this book is neither directive nor non-directive; rather it is a facilitating approach. Facilitating in the sense that the professional helper works with the young person to identify the young person's thoughts, feeling and behaviours; to help them to develop the skills which will enable them to take charge of their own decisions and actions *in the context of their own lives.*

In contrast, a directive approach implies that the helper takes charge of what happens to the young person; thus the helper's attitudes, thoughts and feelings become a central part of the process, and their expert judgements form the basis of what the young person should or should not do.

A non-directive approach in counselling is the opposite of the directive approach in that the counsellor ensures that their attitudes, thoughts and

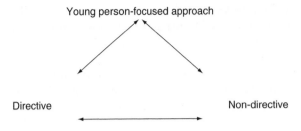

Figure 5.1 The young person-focused approach.

feelings do not impinge on the client in any way. The non-directive counsellor does not facilitate in any specific sense. For example, it would be perfectly acceptable to sit with the client without talking for the whole session, if that was what the client wished. A non-directive approach works towards the goal of self-improvement but would not intervene in that process.

The young person-focused approach as used in professional helping, rather than clinical therapy, is not a half-way position between the directive and non-directive approaches to helping as figure 5.1 illustrates. It is an alternative to either of these models of helping and works toward negotiated goal and action-orientated behaviour.

The young person-focused approach is appropriate for a wide range of helping purposes and settings. The approach fits well with the range of theoretical approaches that the professional helper can draw on and integrate into their applied model. This fit is illustrated further in two well-known introductions to counselling that we referred to previously: Nelson-Jones (2005) and Egan (2002). Both writers demonstrate in different ways the links between a person-centred approach, the range of helping situations and the psychological theories that inform such work.

Another important aspect of a young person-focused approach, because of the various points that have been made so far, is flexibility. A young person-focused approach should be flexible and adaptable to the needs and context of the individual and the demands of the situation. Egan in particular stresses the need for flexibility, in not adhering to a formula of predetermined procedures. As he suggests, a helping model is a framework and his particular model is participative for both the person seeking help and the helper. The process Egan describes is based on a view that to be effective the helper needs to be aware not only of the needs of the client, but also self-aware in order to recognise when the structure, and their own values, are getting in the way of skilled helping.

So far, we have looked at methods of helping and in particular the person-centred model of helping. The positive orientation of the helper towards the young person, including their attitudes, thoughts and feelings about the young person, has been stressed. In addition to these, the competent helper needs a range of skills and strategies in order to facilitate effectively. The range of skills and strategies is outlined in chapter 6; however, it is relevant at this point to highlight again the importance of listening skills for the young person-focused approach. For the approach to be non-prescriptive, the young person's thoughts, feelings and ideas need to be placed centre stage. It is crucial that the helper listens carefully and really hears what the young person is saying. This does, of course, form part of the empathetic role proposed by Rogers.

To take this further, we also need to recognise that for certain groups or individuals expressing these thoughts, feelings and ideas can be difficult. It may be that the individual is not used to articulating these in a style that 'suits' us; or it may be an uncharacteristic activity for the individual, or not part of their culture to consider *individual* thoughts, feeling and needs. To be non-prescriptive is also not easy when the young person expects you to tell them what to do, and there may be times when a direct intervention is appropriate. What may appear a natural approach to us, may not feel natural for the young person – hence the need for a flexible approach and the need to draw on a range of theoretical models.

However, the aim of this book is to give readers one helpful framework as a starting point! As reflective practitioners, readers will want to build on this framework with a range of strategies taken from other models and approaches as they develop in their helping role (some of these are included in the annotated reading list). Of course, none of us enter learning situations as 'empty slates' and many helpers will already have relevant experience and skills, which they will adapt for new working contexts. In adopting any counselling model, whether a person-centred model or some other, the practitioner has to develop their own style and way of using such a model. Models are not prescriptions but structures designed to help practitioners, to give them the confidence to develop the knowledge and skills that will inform their work. Both Rogers and Egan point to the value of 'being oneself' and of sharing the helping process with those seeking help. In order to do this effectively the helper needs to understand the process thoroughly, so that they can explain it to the young person in a way that can be easily understood and valued.

Sharing the process and working alongside the young person helps them to contribute more actively and to understand the relevance of what is happening. Not sharing the process, because the helper does not know why they are doing what they are doing, is not only unhelpful for the young person, but also makes it difficult for the helper to identify what works and what does not. Not sharing with the young person because they would not understand, or because the helper has a reluctance to divulge 'trade secrets', is not congruent with the desire to work towards an equal relationship between the young person and the helper.

To conclude this section, what we have outlined are the principles of the person-centred or young person-focused approach. You will find it valuable to read further about this and other models of helping, to assist you to develop a framework that you can apply to your own role as a professional helper. There is a sizable literature on counselling skills and approaches that has relevance for the work. Some of these are included in the reference list.

The outcomes of helping

Definition:

> *The benefits gained by the young person because of their engagement with the helping process, in respect of meeting their needs.*

The outcomes of helping are the results of seeking assistance with known and unknown helping or guidance needs. These outcomes are very difficult to measure, and the issues can be followed up in more detail by referring to the work of John Killeen (1996).

The outcomes of helping are what young people want as a result of using an agency, professional helper, or a friend or relative who is acting in the capacity of helper. For example, a young person wants help with making a decision (need = decision making skills). The result, that is the outcome of helping, should be that the young person has acquired decision making skills. The young person is now able to make and implement a decision as an outcome of the help they have received. Therefore, in order for the help to be judged effective, the young person must have moved forward from their starting point, that is the point they were at before they sought and used professional help. The outcomes of helping can therefore be seen as a measure of what has been achieved as a result of the helping process.

Ideally, outcomes should be definable and measurable so that the young person is able to recognise and acknowledge the value of the help they have received. Measurable outcomes are also essential to the professional helper so that they can reflect on how effective, or otherwise, the help they have offered has been for the young person. In other words, outcomes are valuable feedback for both the young person and helper but, most importantly, outcomes that enable the young person to manage change and make decisions are the *raison d'être* of the helping process.

There are four generally accepted elements, which young people need in order to make effective decisions. These are:

- self-awareness – young people need to understand their situation and know what they are like, and what they want;
- opportunity-awareness – young people need to know what options are open to them, currently and for the future;
- decision making skills – young people need to know how to approach making decisions appropriately, and how to plan;

- transition skills – young people need to know what may be involved in a transition and how to implement plans.

The above is sometimes known as the DOTS model – a useful mnemonic based on the initial letters, although in a different sequence to that presented above. The above order is probably the most effective in terms of developing young people's thinking about their next steps. These steps have since been reworked and extended by Bill Law (1996): however there is some elegance in the simplicity of the original DOTS model for those new to this work.

Professional helpers often find that their approach to young people becomes much more focused as they begin to think about what young people are actually getting from the help given. In fact they become much more young person-focused. This does not make our work easier as we recognise that each young person has individual needs, but it does make it more stimulating and interesting, and it is easier to help young people who are motivated to succeed. This motivation happens if young people can see for themselves that what is offered will meet their needs.

The range of appropriate outcomes will vary according to the nature and purpose of the help offered. The following examples could apply to a wide range of helping relationships in different helping contexts.

Positive outcomes – the young person:

- has greater self-awareness;
- has an understanding of possibilities;
- has begun to evaluate possibilities;
- has recognised decisions need to be made;
- has begun to formulate decisions;
- is aware of their information needs and how these can be met;
- has begun to evaluate information;
- has begun to formulate/has formulated an action plan;
- has begun to implement their action plan;
- now feels confident about managing change in their life;
- is aware of other agencies or sources of help that might be relevant;
- has acquired decision making skills;
- recognises further needs they may need help with.

As is apparent from this list of possible outcomes, a number of them do not relate to ultimate goals (for example, 'a well-paid job that I will really love'), but do reflect outcomes that might be achieved along the way, as the young person moves through the helping process (for example, 'I'm able to list my strengths and my interests').

We have talked about the advantages, to both professional helper and young person, of being able to measure the outcomes of the helping relationship. Some outcomes are much easier to measure than others. For example, if a young person makes and implements a decision as a result of seeking help from a professional helper, this could be identified as an outcome of the helping process. However, if, as a result of engaging in a helping relationship, a young person increases their self-confidence, it is much more difficult to attribute this to the helping process, as there could be other factors influencing this. We introduced the notion of 'soft outcomes' in the previous chapter, here we draw on Dewson *et al.* (2000) who identify a fuller list of examples:

> [These are] outcomes from training, support or guidance interventions, which unlike hard outcomes, such as qualifications and jobs, cannot be measured directly or tangibly. *Soft outcomes* may include achievement relating to:
>
> - Interpersonal skills, for example: social skills and relating to authority
> - Organisational skills, such as: personal organisation, and the ability to order and prioritise
> - Analytical skills, such as: the ability to exercise judgement, managing time or problem solving, and
> - Personal skills, for example: insight, motivation, confidence, reliability and health awareness.
>
> (Dewson *et al.* 2000: 2)

Frequently these soft outcomes are of great importance to the young person, but are difficult to measure, and are therefore often overlooked, particularly in the context of justifying a service: it is much easier to count numbers of young people helped, than to consider the qualitative impact of the help provided to young people. It is possible to find ways of showing 'soft outcomes' in order to help justify a service. This involves establishing a 'baseline' – or starting point from which individual achievement can be measured, and establishing 'distance travelled' – how far the individual has progressed in achieving the outcomes (Dewson *et al.* 2000).

Exercise: measuring soft outcomes

From your own experience or observation of practice, can you think of a situation where a young person has 'moved on' and achieved 'soft outcomes' as a result of working with a professional helper? What was the 'baseline' – the issue at the starting point – and what was the 'distance travelled' – the outcome? How was this achieved?

Effective helping

All the helping activities and interventions that contribute to the helping process rely on a range of effective interactions. To be effective, these interactions will not depend on just the helper's interpersonal skills, important though these are. The helper will also draw upon their knowledge of theory and practice relating to the lives of young people, their understanding of policies and developments at both a national and local level, and so forth. The helper will use their knowledge, understanding, skills and resources in a wide range of interactions and activities that form helping provision.

In this way, these aspects of the helping process, helping activities and interventions are linked with effective interactions, which are looked at in detail in what follows. The integrated helping model (SIM) attempts to identify and examine key elements that appear to be common to purposeful interactions. Although it is impossible to segregate these elements, seven of these are defined and considered in detail. That said, it is *NOT* a checklist. It is critical to understand that this is not a recipe of essential ingredients, but a recognition of appropriate aspects that must be used *flexibly* in order to meet the needs of the young person and the demands of the situation. The definitions here are offered as additional 'tools to think with' in your work with young people.

The seven elements are:

- young person;
- process;
- skills;
- content;
- issues;
- strategies;
- positive outcomes.

These elements are now examined briefly.

1 The young person

Definition:

> *The individual seeking help from a professional helper.*

We need to recognise that each person has unique experiences, emotions, skills, expectations, resources, behaviours, relationships and tolerances: these ask for understanding and require the professional helper to make as few assumptions as possible. A helper's approach needs to demonstrate adaptability and spontaneity, therefore providing unique solutions to individual needs.

Frequently young people, as we have seen before, are dealing with a range of issues, as a result of the stage of development they are 'at' when we are working with them. Coleman and Hendry (1999) have studied young people's situations in the context of their 'whole' lives, and identified a wide range of factors to consider:

- physical development;
- thinking and reasoning;
- the self and identity;
- families;
- adolescent sexuality;
- adolescent health;
- friendship and peer groups;
- work, unemployment and leisure;
- young people and anti-social behaviour;
- politics, altruism and social action;
- stress coping and adjustment.

Coleman and Hendry (1999) suggest that many young people manage adolescence without too much difficulty, as they are dealing with these issues one at a time. For those who have a more difficult time, it may be because too many of the issues are coming 'into focus' at once, so there is too much to deal with. The 'focal model' Coleman and Hendry put forward seeks to explain this. As helpers, we are likely to be working with young people who are having difficulties in some aspect of their lives, so we need to be aware of the possible impact this may have. It is important to see young people in this holistic context, not just in the light of the issue they may seek help with.

2 The process of effective helping

Definition:

The basic stages through which the helping relationship moves.

This should be a flexible route, rather like a road map in that the appropriate starting points and destinations vary for each 'journey', and the 'route' will depend on the young person's current situation, needs and skills. The process will not always start at the same point, not always take the same route, nor will it necessarily follow the most direct route. However, even if not linear, it does aim to make progress.

The three basic stages are:

- **Opening**   The helper seeks to establish with the young person the purpose of the helping relationship and their perception of it, in order to agree appropriate objectives.
- **Development**   Opportunities are provided for the young person to focus, explore, clarify and address ideas and issues relevant to them. The discussion is renegotiated appropriately in order to maintain relevance. Appropriate goals will be identified and set.
- **Action and conclusion**   Where goals have been identified and set, the helper will enable the young person to identify action that will help them to achieve their goals. The process is concluded with a summary to reflect what has been discussed, agreed as a result of the discussion, and action to be taken following the interaction (you should by now recognise this as the three-stage Single Interaction Model of helping).

3 The skills

Definition:

> *Behaviour and use of language, both verbal and non-verbal, appropriate to effective helping.*

Skills should be analysed in tandem with the process of an effective helping relationship, because some of these skills will be more appropriate at certain stages and less so at others. In addition, skills need to be used flexibly and adapted to the context and to the young person. The following is a bank of skills and qualities or attitudes, that can be drawn on as appropriate to the situation:

Active listening	Questioning	Clarifying	Demonstrating
Reflecting	Paraphrasing	Drawing threads	acceptance
Negotiating	Summarising	Challenging	Understanding
Making links	Immediacy	Empathy	Honesty
			Openness

The skills will be considered in more detail in the next chapter. In addition, both Egan (2002) and Nelson-Jones (2005) have written at some length about the skills needed, in a counselling context, to work effectively with 'clients'.

4 The content

Definition:

> *The identification of appropriate subject matter in relation to the needs of the young person.*

Through the appropriate use of the skills listed above, the helper becomes more sensitive to those ideas and issues that are uniquely important to each young person. The way that the young person is perceived to view the world should not be dependent on an inflexible checklist approach.

5 The issues

Definition:

> *Ideas and concerns which require deeper examination and clarification in order for helping to be effective.*

Issues could be related to needs, values, fears or aspirations, and could be influenced by the factors considered by Coleman and Hendry (1999). Issues should not be confused with problems. Most young people will have issues that they could work on with a professional helper: for example subject choices or managing their time, which they do not necessarily consider to be problems. Some will have real problems, such as experiencing sustained bullying or homelessness, and will need more intensive help and support. That said, it is important to remember that positive ideas, for example choosing between two offers of a job, may need as much attention for some young people as perceived difficulties.

This element of helping recognises not only that different young people may have different priorities, but that each individual young person will have their own unique issues. For example, not all young people in Year 11 will believe that considering their 'next steps' is a critical issue, and for some young people fitting in with a group of peers may be more important than individual choices related to education, training or employment.

6 Strategies

Definition:

> *Effective methods for coping with and assisting young people in addressing the issues to be dealt with.*

Again, although similar issues may be important to different young people, the strategies for assisting may differ because of the individual young person's own skills, experiences and circumstances. The use of strategies, however, will enable the helper and the young person to cope more effectively. Examples of issues that may benefit from specific strategies include:

- decision making;
- clarifying preferences and priorities;
- generating ideas;
- identifying advantages and disadvantages.

There are many more. Some of these can be dealt with effectively within a systematic method that provides a clear structure, which helps both the young person and helper to grasp the task. There are a number of methods or problem solving techniques that can be used to help young people deal with ideas and issues – many are discussed in the next chapter.

7 Positive outcomes

Definition:

> *The recognition of benefits gained by the young person as a result of the interaction.*

In order for the interaction to be effective, the young person must have moved forward from their starting point. In recognising this, the helper and young person are both reinforcing these benefits and acknowledging the value of the service that they have received. The possible outcomes are many and varied, and are dealt with in some detail in an earlier section of this chapter.

The seven elements are closely interrelated, and are dependent on one another for the success of the model in practice. Helping is a complex process, and an awareness of the various strands within it can enable practitioners to be more effective in their helping relationships with young people.

Summary

This chapter has spent some time 'unpacking' the young person-centred approach through an exploration of outcomes, evaluation and the aspects that work towards making helping effective. In undertaking that analysis, we have warned against taking a singular 'world view' and highlighted the insufficiencies of considering only objective measurements for positive outcomes. The chapter has also cautioned against following a rigid structure when framing helping interactions. Structure is important but needs to be flexible: it is our view that both process and skills are interdependent. The next chapter moves on and looks at the skills and strategies that make the process 'come alive' – in practice.

6 Helping skills and strategies

Introduction

The previous chapters have provided the background, or foundation, to enable us to move on to look at helping skills and strategies. In this chapter we will be looking at the range of communication and interpersonal skills that a helper needs, in order to be effective when working with young people in a range of settings. Much of the material covered may be familiar to you depending on your own experience and background, so what you read will in many cases confirm or review what you already know – this should be reassuring! On the other hand, this might be the first time that you have thought about the communication skills that you already have and their professional application to your current role. If the latter is the case, then you will want to do some additional reading, to add to the ideas that are introduced in this chapter. Also in this chapter we will consider a range of strategies that are useful in a helping context.

Verbal and non-verbal communication

We are all skilled and sophisticated communicators. However, the fact that we use these skills in our everyday as well as our professional lives means that we tend to take these skills for granted. We may not give communication skills a great deal of thought or detailed attention, yet they are essential for any 'working with people' job and especially so for youth support work.

We communicate with both spoken and body language, that is verbal and non-verbal behaviour: what follows offers a categorisation of verbal and non-verbal communication:

Verbal communication

Dimension	Example
Volume	Loudness, quietness, audibility.
Tone	Enthusiasm, anger, calmness, disinterest.

Pitch	High, low.
Clarity	Good enunciation, mumbling.
Pace	Fast, slow, even, uneven.

Non-verbal communication

Dimension	Example
Proximity	Closeness, distance, ability to touch.
Posture	Leaning forwards or backwards. Tense, rigid, relaxed. Facing, turned away.
Facial expression	Expressive, blank, smiling, frowning.
Gaze	Staring, avoiding, eye contact.
Gesture	Amount, variety.
Touch	Intimate, aggressive, avoidance.

Non-verbal messages are powerful and can indicate thoughts and feelings that are not congruent with the verbal message. For example, a young person who says 'I could try to go to the college open day', whilst looking away or troubled, is unlikely to be committed to this action. The verbal message is 'I will try', the non-verbal message is 'but I'll fail'. Paying attention to the non-verbal message, we would ask, 'You say you will try but I'm picking up that it may be difficult. What would stop you going?' It may be that the young person does not know where the college is, is not confident to go alone, does not like using public transport or is simply not interested enough.

Of course, whilst watching the young person's body language we also need to be aware of the messages we send via our own body language. And, as argued earlier, we need to be aware that body language varies across groups and cultures. In other words, the same gesture, for example avoiding eye contact, may convey a different meaning to different groups. Along with an understanding of the use of body language, practitioners need a range of interpersonal skills that they can use in a variety of ways with the young people they work with. These are looked at in detail below.

Attending and listening skills

Attending and listening skills are fundamental for effective helping to take place and their importance cannot be over-emphasised. We have all experienced the feeling that we 'have not been listened to' at some time. This may make us feel dismissed, misunderstood or not accepted and can affect our self-esteem, as well as our confidence about our thoughts and feelings. It is crucial that this does not happen to the young people we work with, whatever level of help they require. One of the most important ways of being young person-focused is to listen, in the most active way possible, to what they have to say.

Applying listening skills

Both Rogers and Egan talk about listening skills in counselling contexts, and both stress the value and quality of listening and attending in order to establish an effective working relationship with the 'client'. These skills are relatively easy to describe but require practice to use effectively. We are not good listeners automatically, or good helpers simply because we care and want to help. Time spent acquiring and developing your active listening skills will be of immense value for all your work with young people, and with colleagues in other settings. But what does active listening and attending look like? If you have an opportunity to observe an experienced practitioner you should be able to 'see' the following:

- Verbal following: the use of comments that follow directly from what the speaker is saying. This is perhaps the most difficult listening skill to acquire. It involves allowing the young person to speak without interruption, following what is being said by asking related questions and making comments, without changing the subject or expressing judgments. You thus 'reflect back' what the young person has said to demonstrate understanding, to gain clarification and to acknowledge that you are really hearing what is being said. You also stay with the young person's agenda rather than moving on too quickly to what you think is more important.
- Non-verbal aspects of attending and listening: demonstrated through facial expression, tone of voice, gaze, gestures, posture and physical proximity. Non-verbal communication can help to complete or elaborate the verbal utterances, can signal 'turn taking' in interactions and give other feedback signals to the speaker and listener. Non-verbal listening and attending demonstrates attention and understanding, agreement or surprise, mainly through facial expression; for example, position of the mouth, eyebrows, and via nods, leaning forward, eye contact and para-verbal signals, for instance, the use of 'hmm, yeah' and other sounds.
- Posture: adopting an open and relaxed posture. This gives the impression of being relaxed and having an open mind, which in turn can help to put the young person at ease.

Bearing in mind what has been said previously about culture-specific body language, it is interesting to note the following:

- Reinforcement: in an interaction involving two people, each person 'looks' for 50 per cent of the time, but 'mutual gaze' occupies only about 25 per cent of the time, during 'looking while talking'. This takes the form of glances that usually last about three seconds and mutual glances of about one second; rather than sustained staring.

Exploration and clarification skills

Apart from showing our understanding with our non-verbal behaviour, we enhance our listening and understanding with responses that help to explore and clarify the issues under discussion. This also helps us to agree priorities with the young person and to see the issues within their frame of reference. We achieve this through our use of questioning, employing the techniques of:

- reflecting;
- probing and prompting;
- checking and clarifying.

Questioning techniques

Exploration and clarification will involve the use of questions. There are several types of question, all of which are used in interactions. However, different questions demand varying types of responses, so they are used in different ways, to make the discussion more effective. Here is a brief outline of question types:

- Open questions: these are questions that are difficult to answer with just 'yes' or 'no'. They give the young person the opportunity to explain the issue and to describe their thoughts, feelings and experiences. Open questions tend to begin with 'how', 'what', 'where', and may include 'why' questions; although care needs to be taken with 'why', as it can be over-challenging for some young people if used too early in the relationship. 'Why?' can sound like 'Come on – justify yourself!' Using the right tone of voice with 'Tell me what' or 'Tell me how' is more collaborative than 'Why do you?' questions. But there is a place for 'why' questions and, when used, 'why' can be softened and becomes more collaborative by asking 'I'm wondering why' or 'Tell me why'. Of course 'Tell me' is not a question and therefore is less 'testing': it creates an opening, as it is an invitation rather than a command for information.
- Closed questions: in contrast to open questions, closed questions tend to demand 'yes' or 'no' answers. They begin with 'do you', 'have you', 'would you', 'can you' and so on. If a young person is shy or reticent then the safest answer is 'no', to close down the questioning and avoid giving a 'wrong' answer. Closed questions are useful if you need a straight 'yes' or 'no' answer. Open questions are better for exploration and too many closed questions may make the young person feel that they are being interrogated.
- Leading questions: these suggest that the helper already knows the answer and the young person may find it hard to disagree. Therefore they are very limiting, if not misleading, and are best avoided. You might like to observe how often people use leading questions in their

conversations, for example, 'you don't like lots of new things happening at once, do you?' It can be a difficult habit to break and we are often unaware that we are 'leading' and therefore 'putting words in other people's mouths'. With every leading question there comes a value judgement on behalf of the helper that does not 'fit' with a young person-focused approach.

- Multiple questions: these confuse people by demanding several responses at once, and they do not know which to answer first. They are definitely to be avoided. A variation is 'marathon questions'; these are so long that by the time the question has ended no one (including the helper) really knows what it was about!
- Double questions: present only two 'either/or' choices, but can still be confusing and restrict instead of widening options, so are best avoided unless used to help the young person compare and contrast ideas.
- Hypothetical questions: these are useful to help a young person to think about and 'envision' a possible option or goal, or the implications of that goal for their circumstances. They often start with 'If you were . . . what . . .'.
- Supplementary questions: these reflect back, so they rely on listening well to be effective. They are useful for clarification.
- Restatement: this is a summary in a questioning form or tone that helps to reflect the young person's comments back to them, in order to check understanding.

Exercise – Listening skills

You can experience the effects of active listening and helpful questioning skills by trying out the following with a friend or colleague.

1 Using body language that demonstrates a lack of genuine interest and acceptance, ask about your partner's dream holiday, give little feedback, interrupt and talk about your dream holiday. Ask your partner how that felt.
2 This time using positive body language, listen, ask open questions, encourage further development with 'say more about' and stay with your partner's dream holiday. When closed questions are used the 'rule' for this exercise is to answer with 'yes', 'no' or 'dunno'! Identify with your partner how the second experience differed from the first.
3 Swap so that you both get to experience ineffective and effective communication skills!

One thing that needs to be used in conjunction with helpful questioning and active listening is *silence*. Using silence in a sensitive manner can encourage the young person to take time to respond to your question, to gather their thoughts and expand a little further. In normal conversation, or when we are feeling anxious, we give people around four seconds to respond to us before we 'jump in', to either answer our own question, or to move on to something else. Four seconds is an inadequate amount of thinking time for responding to questions about ourselves; questions which may be quite challenging or thought provoking. It takes experience and confidence to resist the temptation to rescue the young person in these circumstances. Rather than 'leap in', if the young person is struggling too much, it will be more fruitful to think about the question that you just asked. Take the blame and rephrase, for example, 'Maybe that wasn't very clear so let me put that another way', or 'I didn't express that very well, let me try again.'

Rapport-building skills

In a collaborative approach, where the aim is to work alongside the young person, it is essential that the young person and the helper have a comfortable working relationship. In other words, an effective working relationship means there is openness and trust. It is important that the helper establishes a constructive and productive relationship using a number of rapport-building skills. These skills create the atmosphere and set the tone. It is important to create the right atmosphere so that both parties can work together effectively. When there are time constraints rapport needs to be established quickly, so this is an important and fundamental skill.

The following identifies the skills and behaviours that demonstrate effective rapport-building:

- Helper's self-presentation: the initial welcome and the introduction of self, that is, name, title or role. This should be friendly and sincere. The importance of the helper's self-presentation does, of course, continue to be crucial for maintaining rapport throughout the interaction and will be displayed by interest, attention, warmth, respect, empathy, congruence, sincerity and so on.
- Introductions: these are important to establish the reason for both parties being present. This may be as simple as ensuring that the young person knows who you are. Spending time (sharing understanding rather than 'telling them') on the beginning of the interaction in terms of introductions, purpose and what might be gained, are vital for building rapport with the young person and for getting the working relationship established. We will be looking at the beginnings of one-to-one interactions in more detail in the final chapter.

- Verbal and non-verbal communication: helps to create and maintain rapport. All the dimensions of communication that we looked at earlier – tone, eye contact, posture and so on – will either enhance or undermine rapport between the young person and the helper.

Using the young person's name during the discussion is an obvious way of maintaining rapport. Another useful point to bear in mind is to avoid the continuous use of 'you', as in 'What do you need to do/think about?' Using 'we' is more involving, and using 'other people', as in 'I'm wondering, what do other people do/think?', can take the pressure off the intensity of using 'you' all the time.

So, the helper needs to be observant and sensitive to the impact that they are having on the young person and adjust their approach accordingly. The young person may be shy, quiet, talkative, verbose, hesitant, reluctant, withdrawn, resentful or over-eager. The helper needs to be able to communicate effectively, and have a good working relationship with each and every young person, regardless of the issues they bring and the manner in which they present themselves.

Of course for some young people requiring intensive support, the time spent on rapport building may be considerable and cannot be rushed. But learning to build trust with the professional helper will be a valuable learning experience for them, and once achieved will help the practitioner and the young person to move on to develop goals and action.

Summarising

Summaries 'sum up' ideas, thoughts and feelings. However, in helping interactions, summaries are not just used as ending points or conclusions. Summaries can and should be used throughout the discussion. Like focusing, summaries can help the young person and helper to gain a sense of direction. Summaries also 'reflect' to the young person what they have said, what you have discussed together and the agreed action to be taken. Providing this opportunity for the young person to hear what they have said can be powerful. It leads to deeper thought within the interaction; for example, 'Did I say that – is that what I really think?' Summaries, like other helping skills, are used as part of the collaborative process – talking with a shared purpose – and benefit both helper and young person.

Summaries can be a very useful tool prior to focusing – look again at figure 2.3 (page 20). Summaries are a means of drawing the initial, exploratory discussion together, and identifying clearly appropriate issues for further discussion. Summaries can help the practitioner to present the issues that will assist both parties to be clear about where to start, or where to go next, and thus clarify the focus and direction for the remainder of their work together.

Again, this process may need to be repeated in an individual interaction as new ideas and issues emerge. Summaries can provide an opportunity to re-negotiate the content of the discussion, which helps to maintain flexibility and avoid rigidity. Summaries can also help when you 'lose the thread'. If you are not sure where an interaction is going, the young person is probably also unsure. A summary will help to get you both back on course. If you are really lost, use honesty/be congruent and say, 'I've lost the plot a bit here, what did we say earlier . . . or how did we get to this point . . .?' – this provides a good opportunity to re-engage the young person and emphasises the collaborative nature of the work. At any subsequent meeting with the young person, in the initial stage of the interaction, it is logical and helpful to begin with a short summary of the previous work and a review of any agreed action.

Getting the skill of summarising right is not easy. When you first use this skill it will seem that you are merely repeating what has just been said and you will question its usefulness. Persevere and you will move from repetition to reflective summarising skills that will help you both to clarify understanding, achieve focus, 'signpost' what has been achieved and what happens next and move forward to shared action.

Advanced skills for exploration, evaluation and action planning

The skills already discussed provide the foundation for a collaborative working relationship and are used throughout the stages of the work. Moving on, the skills of information sharing and challenging are often described as advanced skills: they are essential for the exploration in Stage 2 of the Single Interaction Model and for evaluation and action planning in Stage 3. These stages in the model were introduced in chapter 2 and will be considered in more detail in the final chapter.

The use of information

Sharing information is a valuable helping activity. It is important to remember that informing is simply the provision of information, without any discussion of the relative merits of alternatives. It is not the practitioner's role to decide what is 'good' or 'bad' about opportunities, products, services and so on. However, it *is* the practitioner's role to help the young person to make sense of the information that is available, and this is contained in the helping activity of 'advising' discussed in an earlier chapter. These two helping activities are closely linked, but we need to be aware of their separateness in order that we use them to best advantage. In what follows we will be looking at two specific information activities, **information gathering** and **information sharing**. Each activity forms an important part of the helping process.

Information gathering

Much of the information gathering will take place in the opening stage of the work – which is about initial exploration and clarification. However, we need to continue information gathering throughout the work with a young person, as further issues and ideas emerge. It is very easy to ask the young person many questions and gather lots of information: the result is likely to be confusion for both you and them. To be effective we need to be clear about *what* information we need and *why* we need it and, in addition, we need to be mindful of data protection issues. If you do not have a clear purpose in mind when you are seeking information then perhaps you should be asking yourself why you are collecting it.

Information sharing

'Sharing' means a two-way process where both parties contribute. It is important to remember this so that you do not ignore one of the most significant resources you have, the young person. What do they already know, what access to further information do they have? They may have information that you are not aware will be helpful. Sharing information, as you work alongside the young person, will help you to build a clear and full picture. It is important to enable the young person to contribute whenever possible and not to overlook, and in so doing, dismiss what they already know.

When asking questions here, look for the 'spark' or 'hook' that will get the young person engaged. In other words, explore the interest first with 'Tell me more about . . .' questions and avoid the rush into exploring what else they need to know. And, try to avoid the 'What do you know about . . .' question (often repeated): although open, this begins to sound like a test and is not collaborative. On the receiving end it sounds like, 'I'm the expert and I know, but I'm going to test how much you know.'

One of the most important rules of information sharing, or providing information, is not to pretend that you have information that you do not. If you genuinely do not know something, it is vital to be honest. There is no disgrace in not knowing everything, but there is in pretending you do: far better to admit that you do not know, suggest it would be good to agree what precise information is needed and then talk about ways of finding out. For example a response might be, 'I'm not sure and I don't want to give you misleading information, let's think about what we need to know precisely and how we could find out together.'

When discussing information gathering and information sharing, we also need to be clear about confidentiality and its limits, and ensure that this is discussed with the young person. By the same token, we have already stated that they should also be involved in the decision relating to any referral to another helper or agency.

Sharing information effectively

Information is a tool – it can be used as a means of helping a young person to move forward in their thinking. But information is a means, not an end! Its value is not in what you know or how much you know: its worth comes from the *way* in which you use it, the way in which it is applied. We must be careful not to bombard or deluge young people with information. It is very easy to clutch on to what we feel we know and regurgitate it at every opportunity. When this happens the information we give is often inappropriate, and although it may make us feel secure it rarely meets the young person's needs.

Sharing information effectively is an activity that is undertaken together, something you both participate in; it is a two-way discussion, a dialogue. Because it is shared it is assumed that you will both have something to contribute. You are helping the young person to *add* to what they *already* know so as to equip them for taking responsibility for their next step. You can pool your joint knowledge in order to address issues that you have identified together – you share your knowledge.

As tutors observing the use of guidance skills, we have both been in situations working with novice practitioners when we have seen the helper 'glow' as they realise that the 'client' wants information about something they, the helper, know lots about. One example was an education adviser who was asked about a university degree in geography. The adviser had undertaken this degree a few years previously, and with great enthusiasm told the client all about it. After a fairly long 'speech' the helper sat back, rather pleased with this information giving, inviting a response from the client. The client, looking peeved, responded with, 'Yes, I know all that, thanks!' The helper had not 'pooled' their joint knowledge and had not paid attention to the client's withdrawn body language.

Exercise – information sharing

To practise the advanced skill of information sharing you could try the following with a colleague:

1 First create a scenario where you as the helper can answer questions about a service, training/education opportunity or career that you know a lot about. Now tell your partner all about it – fill them up with your knowledge and expertise.
2 Pick another topic that you are an 'expert' on. This time hold back and share information, finding out what your partner knows first, how they know that, explore what the gaps in their knowledge might be and discuss this with them. You can use your knowledge, but share rather than overwhelm.
3 Discuss both approaches. Again, it is useful to swap so that you experience this from both sides.

Discovering information

Ideally, young people should be enabled to discover information for themselves, whenever this is appropriate. This will help them to feel a sense of ownership in the information seeking process, which for many young people can help them to feel motivated and open to absorbing the ideas or facts contained in the information. This also helps to avoid information being imposed on them by the helper. When we are adding to a young person's knowledge, with information that we have both agreed is relevant to their needs, we are helping them to see things in a new light and equipping them to make decisions – however small.

Information can be quite challenging for a young person. They may discover that what they want to do next has unexpected implications, good or bad, or that a service they thought would be available is not. For example, the latter could be anything from free transport to being provided with a flat of their own. This discovery could be motivating or experienced as a barrier. Young people, depending on their circumstances and needs, will require your support to interpret the information: to explore the implications and relevance for their context.

In addition, the way we provide information when working one-to-one is important, just as important as it is with information gathering. We need to:

- check the young person's understanding of what they are being told or are discovering;
- seek their opinion as to how the information can be applied;
- be aware of how the young person is responding to what they are discovering (are they looking awkward, deflated, confused, angry, interested or involved? What do they feel about what they are finding out?);
- avoid overwhelming the young person with information. If we give too much, too soon it will be indigestible. Five minutes after they leave it will be as if you had never told them.

Bombarding young people with information pushes them out of the discussion. If they have to sit quietly and listen to you for too long, they will 'switch off' (if you undertook the exercise above it is likely you experienced this feeling). This may reflect their prior experience: in other words they may think that this is appropriate behaviour, they are there to 'shut up and be told'. Information should be shared and the young person needs to be involved actively in this. Information gathering/information sharing sounds easy, but it is an advanced skill that requires practice in order to be used effectively and in a collaborative manner.

Challenging

The aim of challenging is to help the young person to gain a new perspective or increased awareness of a particular idea, thought, behaviour or feeling. This can help the young person to identify ways in which they are being prevented, or are preventing themselves, from reaching goals; and can also help them to gain a better understanding of themselves and their situation.

Challenging is a constructive 'confrontation' that needs to be handled sensitively by the helper, so that it aids reflection on 'faulty thinking' about ideas, feelings and actions in order to help the young person move forward and to make progress. The skill of challenging effectively is one that is acquired with experience. Challenging must be used with great care as a badly handled challenge can do more harm than good. Egan (2002) says that practitioners need to 'earn the right to challenge', and that challenging too soon in the relationship will damage rapport and destroy trust. Challenging can be achieved through an open question, a follow-up question, reflecting back a word or phrase, a summary, use of a hypothetical question, through the use of empathy, through sharing information and through appropriate self-disclosure.

Immediacy is also a challenging skill but is used for a different purpose. We would normally challenge a young person about what they are saying in regard to their thoughts, feelings and actions to issues outside of the interaction. We would use immediacy when something is wrong within the interaction. For example, a young person has been desperate to see you, but when you meet they are withdrawn and uncommunicative. Using immediacy we would try to find out what was wrong in the 'here and now', for example, 'I know you were keen to see me, and yet you do not want to talk to me today – I wonder why that is?'

If challenging is a new skill, or a skill you are aware that you avoid because it feels too confrontational, you will want to explore other examples to gain a greater insight into this powerful but most effective tool (see recommended texts in the annotated list). The ultimate aim of challenging a young person is to be helpful, not to make them sit up and take notice, but for them to learn to reflect and self-challenge. Challenging leads to a deeper exploration of the issue or idea and can help the young person and practitioner to focus and move forward.

When challenging a young person in a helping relationship it will be important to keep the following in mind. A challenge needs to be:

- constructive and relevant to the discussion;
- framed in appropriate, clear language;
- well-timed;
- sensitive, but not endlessly tentative or apologetic;
- positive in its effects, not judgmental.

And the aim of challenging must always be kept in mind within a relationship where the helper demonstrates 'unconditional positive regard'. With this in mind, one way of 'softening' a challenge is to use the words 'I'm wondering' at the start. Other useful phrases might include, 'Something I don't quite understand is . . .' or 'Maybe I got this wrong, but earlier you said . . . how does that fit with . . .'. And, if the young person does not understand the relevance of the challenge, then explain, 'The reason I asked that question was because . . .'.

In the case study that follows, note the way the helper uses both challenge and immediacy, in order to stay with the young person's agenda and to explore the issue in more depth. We pick the interview up in Stage 2, the exploratory stage, after the agenda has been agreed in Stage 1. A quick look at figure 2.1 (page 14) will remind you what each stage covers.

Case study: Jess – 'I'm leaving'

Helper: So Jess, you've talked about what is going on for you at school and you've said you are going to leave home and school and get a flat with a friend. Have I got that right?

Jess: Yes (*sounding defensive*).

Helper: That sounds like an exciting thing to do and yet you don't look or sound excited. I'm picking up that you feel a bit cross at the moment and I'm wondering why that is?

Jess: Well my teacher said I wouldn't get a flat – can you get me one?

Helper: I see, well it may be difficult, certainly, but perhaps we can spend time thinking about what you want and why you want it. If we have a clear picture we can decide what we need to do next, and who we need to talk to. How does that sound?

Jess: Ok, but I'm not gonna change my mind.

Helper: That's fine, as I said earlier my role is to help you explore what the options are and to think about how we can move forward. So, tell me some more about the sort of flat you had in mind.

Jess: Well, I know it won't be huge but we'd like our own bedroom each and a separate TV/sitting area and a small kitchen (*pause*) and a shower room and I'd like it to be in the middle of town, near the shops and station.

Helper: Sounds good, although I'm thinking that may not be the sort of accommodation the agency provides in that area. We'd need to find out, but what if you couldn't get what you want?

continued on next page

Jess: Well (*pause*) I suppose I could look at other places.

Helper: Yeah that could help. Thinking back to what you said a minute ago, tell me why it is important to be near the station?

Jess: (*Silence*)

Helper: (*Waits*)

Jess: I might want to visit my Mum.

Helper: So seeing your Mum would still be important to you Jess?

Jess: Yeah, well, she needs me!

Helper: 'Needs you' – how does that fit, Jess, with your thoughts about leaving?

Jess then begins to talk a little more about the underlying issue of wanting to leave home.

Moving the client forward – some strategies to go with the skills

We can also use strategies to help young people to self-challenge, to sort out their confusion, set priorities or generate new ideas if they are needed. Strategies are very useful for all sorts of issues that young people face, so it is helpful to have a variety of methods to draw on, as some will be more appropriate than others. Strategies form a key part of your 'toolkit' as a helper and, combined with the skills already discussed, will help you to feel well-equipped to deal with a wide range of young people and issues when they are presented to you.

Strategies help the young person to clarify, make sense of, or compare ideas and issues that they need to address, in order to move forward in their thinking. For example, one common strategy is a 'thought-shower' list of possibilities for action. What follows are other ideas that you may already use, or could add to your 'toolkit'.

Imagine

'Imagine' is a very simple strategy. It can provide useful clues about issues that need discussion, in a very short time. It is particularly useful when working with young people who lack confidence or assertiveness, or young people whose ideas are vague or unrealistic.

The technique works like this:

Your young person has talked about things that they would like to change in their life, but so far they have not taken any action. They have been able to find a number of reasons (which appear not very convincing) for not making the changes.

At this point it would be very easy to:

- simply reflect to the young person that they would like to make changes but feel unable to act;
- give the young person information or suggestions about how these changes could be made (this approach shows a lack of acceptance and empathy from the helper and is verging on being directive).

One way forward, to move the young person on in their thinking, is to ask them to imagine that they are making the changes that they have talked about. The young person is asked to describe what it feels like to make the changes and what it is like when the changes have been implemented. The helper may need to use some prompts to get the young person to think about the changes from several perspectives. Using this technique can be quite challenging for a young person when they find that either the envisaged changes are not so drastic as they feared, or the action required to effect change is 'do-able' without too much difficulty.

If the above is not the case, identifying what the problem areas really are, so that these can be discussed and solutions worked on, is itself a move forward. In this way the imagine technique can be a confidence-building exercise, which makes a previously insurmountable problem manageable. Closely related to this technique is the use of the 'miracle question' used in solution focused brief therapy (SFBT) (O'Connell 2001), for example:

> 'If you woke up tomorrow and the problem no longer existed, what would that be like?' followed perhaps by, 'And what would you do next?'

or

> 'If you woke up tomorrow and you could do the course/job of your dreams, what would that course/job be like?'

Contrasts

This technique is particularly helpful for assisting young people with choices, changes or confusion. The main aim is to help the young person gain a better understanding by comparing whatever issue you are focusing on, with something that is significantly different or opposite. This technique often helps the young person to gain a sharper focus.

For example, it may highlight which aspects are really important when choosing future courses of action and making plans. Alternatively, it might help the young person to identify forces that are hindering change and to recognize that these forces are less of a difficulty than not making changes. So, for example, you might ask your young person to a) describe what it will be like to do something that is under consideration and to b) compare and 'contrast' that outcome with not taking any action, so that things do not change and remain as they are as present. Sensitivity and a non-judgmental attitude are, of course, essential here. Alternatively, they can contrast what it would be like to find themselves in two or three different, but possible, scenarios through the use of hypothetical 'If you were' questions. In this way, contrast works a little like the imagine technique but as a means of choosing and/or clarifying.

Gaining figure-ground perspective

This strategy is beneficial when young people are feeling confused or when they are faced with choices and are not sure what to do. The aim of 'gaining figure-ground perspective' is to try and identify the issues or factors that 'stand out' from the rest of the picture, the picture in this case being their 'whole' situation. Initially the young person may present a somewhat muddled picture in which nothing stands out as a major focal point. When you help them place a choice to be made, or a problem to be solved, within a context, and separate the 'figure' (the central issue of concern that figures in the foreground) from the 'ground' (factors around the issue which form the background), you are assisting the young person to gain figure-ground perspective.

To explain this further, imagine you are in an art gallery looking for the first time at a large landscape or seascape painting (for the point of the example, we'll stick with conventional rather than abstract works of art). The painting 'works' when we can get a focus on the story that the painter is depicting. We search for the meaning and a central figure often helps us to access this quickly. Imagine Constable's *The Hay Wain* without the hay wain – lots to look at, but no particular story. When a young person is confused by events in their lives their picture is full of detail, but nothing stands out as the central issue because there is so much to look at, to think about. The background represents their context, and the 'problem' that is stopping them from moving forward could be buried somewhere in the picture. How can you work with them to bring this problem or issue from the background to figure in the foreground? The aim is for the young person to gain a new perspective, which will not be possible until the central issue that is causing a 'problem' has been identified.

To use this technique effectively involves a number of skills. First of all, you will probably need to summarise the situation described by the young person, reflecting what seem to be the issues that have been presented. Once you have checked that your perception of the situation is accurate, and you have agreed the main purpose of the discussion to follow, you will then need to share with the young person what you think the central issue or 'figure' might be. In this way it is rather like 'sharing a hunch', saying what you think might be the case, in a tentative manner to check out whether the young person shares your perception or not. You can then agree whether or not this is a useful way of looking at the situation in order to go forward.

Again, this technique needs to be used sensitively and not applied in order to force a young person to choose arbitrarily one among several things, all of which could be discussed. The main aim is to help the young person separate essential issues from a broad and complex picture, in the middle of which they feel muddled, stuck or 'bogged down'. Also this technique helps you both to look at the 'problem' as something that is separate from them as a person (White and Epston 1990).

Balance sheets

The 'balance sheet' can be used as a decision making tool. It can help a young person to think about the advantages and disadvantages of any ideas or plans that they are considering. It can be used as a method for comparing choices as well as a means of identifying, or increasing awareness of, consequences.

Balance sheets can be very simple, for example two columns headed 'advantages' and 'disadvantages'. The young person is helped by the practitioner to identify what they, the young person, see as advantages and disadvantages in order to assess if one outweighs the other, and to get a balanced picture of the option. If working with a very young person, or with a young person who may have difficulty accepting there may be disadvantages, it can be useful to talk about 'what's really good' and 'what may put some people off'. A more complex balance sheet might involve the pros and cons of two or more options, so that the young person is able to identify the consequences and benefits of each option, and then 'weigh up' and compare the choices.

Force-field analysis

This technique will probably also need pen and paper (and it is worth noting that such exercises, using a pen and paper or whiteboard, can help to relieve any pressure built up through too much eye contact and questioning). The aim of this method is to identify the negative forces (factors related to particular people, circumstances or resources) that constrain a young person from acting or choosing an action, and the positive forces (again, factors related to particular people, circumstances or resources) that will assist them to take action or make a choice (Johnson and Johnson 1994). In other words, what has the young person got 'going for them' and what are the things 'going against them' that are helping or stopping them from achieving their goal? Identifying these positive and negative forces can help both parties to evaluate potential goals and action and helps to work towards action that is more likely to be 'successful'. And remember to join in – again, it's not a test of their knowledge but a strategy to aid joint thinking.

Techniques from solution focused brief therapy

Earlier, reference was made to the miracle question from solution focused brief therapy (SFBT). There are a number of other techniques that can be adapted from SFBT, which are thought to be helpful when working with young people (O'Connell 2001). This book cannot look at the approach in great depth and readers are recommended to follow up the work of O'Connell and others. Other techniques from so-called 'constructivist' approaches, including SFBT and narrative counselling, are included in this chapter. Winslade and Monk (1999) have written a very accessible account of school counselling which combines solution-focused and narrative approaches. Youth support workers who are interested in the approach will find the text helpful. Many of the techniques are simple and practical, and have a pragmatic appeal, but of course they will not work all the time with all young people. So if something does not work, stop doing it, and if something does work, keep on doing it. This is part of the SFBT approach for both the helper in their helping, and for the young person in their current behaviour and future action. Some of the techniques are now described.

Exception seeking

A central theme, indeed the underlying philosophy of constructivist approaches to helping, is the need to separate the person from the problem. This is exemplified in the phrase 'The person isn't the problem; the problem is the problem' (Epston 1989: 26). For example, homelessness is a problem, it is a real issue, not a moral failing on the part of the young person. Homelessness should not define the young person and be the only lens through which they are viewed. Of course, for some young people there will be many problems and issues to deal with. SFBT, like the approach in this book, would stress that urgent issues need to be attended to first. The focus is, however, on what the young person sees as the priority, not what the helper may view as most urgent. Exception seeking asks the young person to describe a time when the issue was not a problem, or was less of a problem. Getting the young person to identify these times can assist both the helper and the young person to think about how that situation can be replicated. This can help to get back a perspective on the issue that is often lost when the young person is feeling overwhelmed by current events.

Scaling

As a strategy for work with young people, scaling can help them to express their thoughts and feelings about issues or problems through the use of numbers. The scale ranges from 0–10, with 0 representing the worst scenario and 10 representing a time when the problem no longer exists. It can help to engage the young person in the evaluation of the current situation and future goals. If a young person describes their current position on the scale as, say, 3, the helper and young person can think together about what needs to happen to raise this to a 4 or 5 and thereby consider what that 4 or 5 would look like.

Do something different

SFBT recognises that when people 'get stuck' in their problems they often repeat behaviour and action that is known (and therefore 'safe'), even when the evidence points to the ineffectiveness of this past behaviour. SFBT would not work to analyse why the behaviour arose, but would look for *agreeable* (in both senses of the word) alternatives to try out. The aim is to work towards more effective action that promotes change. In this way solutions are tried that fit the person, rather than the problem.

Small steps for achievement

Setting small goals can lead to a sense of achievement when these are reached. For many young people who, for whatever reason, do not view themselves as successful, this can be a very positive step in building confidence and self-esteem. The view of self can change from 'I'm a failure' (along with all the potential associated behaviour) to 'I'm a success.'

Compliments

Compliments are 'positive strokes' and enhance the young person's self-concept. As importantly, they encourage ownership in a process where both helper and young person are learning. Compliments can be used in any of the above strategies to reward a young person for something they did in the past, present or are thinking about doing in the future. But, the use of compliments must be genuine or they will sound patronising to both the helper and the young person.

A word of warning! Improper use of these strategies from SFBT can move to action too quickly if inadequate time is spent on the opening steps in Stage 1 of the work, whether this is in a single interaction or as part of a developed professional helping relationship. Although the approach can get a young person moving to action quickly, benefits will not be sustained if the wider context of their lives and 'the problem' is not given due consideration. An outcome-focused approach may fit nicely into a 'what works' agenda, but should not be viewed as an economical way of 'fixing people' quickly. When we 'mine' strategies from counselling models without an understanding of the model's theoretical underpinning, we risk using the skills inappropriately (Reid 2006). To explore the philosophy behind narrative, SFBT and other constructivist approaches, we have included recommended texts in the list at the end of the book (page 111).

Using strategies with young people

To use strategies successfully requires a mixture of familiarity and practise. First, you need to be fairly familiar with the method so that you can use the strategy with a certain degree of confidence; and second, you will need to experiment with using strategies in practice so that you find the ones that you feel most comfortable with. You will be able to find more strategies by talking to your colleagues and by locating the reading in the reference list. Two further examples that we would suggest are very useful for work with young people are, first, the work on motivational interviewing by Rollnick and Miller (1995) and Miller and Rollnick (2002), and second, of particular use for understanding how people communicate, Berne's work on transactional analysis (e.g. 1968).

Of course the strategies and approaches discussed above are not limited to work with young people; they are relevant in a range of settings and with a variety of groups. Finally, using challenging skills, information sharing and exploration strategies can be hard work and the young person will benefit from a reward! A positive stroke or compliment can, as mentioned earlier, be very helpful in the professional relationship. For example:

> I can see that you are really determined, despite the difficulties we've talked about. Thinking about what we said, I'm wondering, what do you think the next step should be?

> You've worked really hard there and we've got a clear picture now of what is going to help and what needs further thought.

Using a challenge or exploration strategy effectively also means knowing when to stop and acknowledging that the young person has the right to withdraw. Of course, you do not use these skills and strategies on their own and will remain attentive to the young person's immediate needs – which may mean 'enough for today'!

Summary

In this chapter we have considered the skills and strategies that need to be developed within a framework for effective helping. We hope that the material has helped you to identify the communication skills that you already have. How we communicate is an important part of our social and professional lives; however, unless we reflect on our use of communication skills it is all too easy to assume that we are effective. Reflection helps us to consider the effects of skills-in-action and to identify those skills we use well, and those skills we need to develop further. This reflection is not just for the novice, it is also part of the continuous professional development of the experienced professional. Part of the joy of the work is experiencing how the effective use of these skills helps the young person to move on, in a way that is meaningful for them and therefore satisfying for you.

The skills and strategies looked at are placed within the young person-focused approach identified in the previous chapter. The next and final chapter looks at the various steps in each stage of the Single Interaction Model.

7 The Single Interaction Model
The helping process

Introduction

In this final chapter we will unpack the structure that helps to frame supportive interventions for work with young people. That structure mirrors the process the young person takes in moving from identifying the problem, exploring the issues and setting goals, to planning and implementing action. The chapter brings together the elements discussed in previous chapters: placing theory, skills and strategies within the suggested framework. Where it repeats points made elsewhere we hope this aids clarification: consolidation is the intention.

Before continuing, it may be helpful to look again at the overview of the model as presented in figures 2.1 and 2.3 (pages 14 and 20). In chapter 2 we discussed the circumstances that would suit the Egan model and/or the Single Interaction Model (SIM). It is not the intention to be prescriptive about this as they are not mutually exclusive – indeed the latter is adapted from the former. Any helping interaction with a young person can follow a simple beginning, middle and end structure (Culley and Bond 2004): SIM helps to articulate short term work whilst Egan is more suited to longer term help. The principles and structures are combined in what follows.

EFFECTIVE HELPING – THE PROCESS – STAGE 1

Stage 1 – current scenario (Egan 2002)
Negotiating the contract and agreeing an agenda (SIM)

A definition of 'the process', which we discussed previously, is:

The basic stages through which the helping relationship moves.

It is this process element of the model that lends the structure and sense of progression to effective helping. Although it sets out the stages that effective helping goes through, it is, however, the antithesis of a checklist. Rather, we have used the metaphor of a map that shows you where you started from, where you hope to get to and roughly where you are on your journey. It requires that you view the young person you are working with as a fellow traveller. Together you plan the route. Such a route may not be the most direct, it may not follow a clear linear progression and may involve some wandering: but it will be the route that is most suitable to the needs of that particular young person. If applied properly, the model acknowledges that all young people are different. It aims to be facilitating, enabling and young person-focused, rather than directive, impersonal and prescriptive.

Stage 1 – opening

Setting the scene, and beginning to clarify and assess the young person's needs, is the initial stage of the meeting. We can identify a number of necessary elements at this stage of the helping relationship. It is important to greet the young person, to introduce ourselves, to check their expectations, to share and explain what we see as the purpose of such a helping relationship (paying attention to ethical issues, such as confidentiality), to establish what they hope to gain from it, to negotiate how far we are able to meet their wishes, to agree a plan for the session and to establish an effective rapport. Such elements, when applied sensibly and flexibly, help to provide the conditions that are necessary for assessing needs and the clarification of issues relevant to the young person.

Central to the assessment of needs and issue clarification is the idea of negotiation and contracting. Contracting is not something that is completed within an opening 'script', but is a theme that runs throughout the work. You are working with the young person, not at them or for them. A contract which agrees ways of working together may need to be renegotiated.

This stage of issue clarification can be broken down further into two steps:

1 **Assessing needs/helping the young person to tell their story.** That is, gaining a clear understanding of the young person's perceptions, and assessing the stage they are 'at' in their thinking about their current situation and their future.
2 **Focusing on the issues that will be addressed in the remainder of the session.** This will be one or two specific issues which, if worked at together, will help the young person to be clearer about their future direction. The helper needs to work with the young person to set specific objectives for the session that are achievable in the time available.

Helping the young person to tell their story

It often takes a while to understand the relevance and importance of Stage 1. The tendency can be to brush over the young person's perceptions and understanding of their own situation, in impatience to make progress and move the young person on. If we do not take time to find out about the young person, and to understand things from their perspective, we are in danger of treating them as a stereotype rather than an individual.

We need to get young people to talk about their ideas, hopes, plans, perceptions, experiences, feelings, uncertainties and enthusiasms. Our role is to observe and listen carefully to the young person, in order to highlight parts of their story that may be useful for the collaborative work ahead. We should help them to describe their situation in relevant and specific terms, with a view to gauging, and verifying with them, where they are in the process of sorting out their ideas. It is helpful to use phrases like, 'Tell me more about . . .' or 'Describe to me how . . .', rather than words like 'explain' or 'why', which ask a young person to justify their views and actions. We need to know how well-informed and 'realistic' they are, but only when we have taken the time to understand young people in an empathic way can we offer effective help.

As we have said previously, the effectiveness of any helping relationship is as dependent on the young person's skills and ability to adapt to the situation, as it is on our own. As such, both parties have tasks to perform which are relevant to this and the steps that follow.

These tasks are, for the helper:

- to exercise the skills and attitudes of listening, attending, prompting, probing and questioning, reflecting back, respect, genuineness and rapport building;

and for the young person:

- to explore the experiences, behaviour and feelings that relate to the issue(s) being discussed in a specific and concrete manner.

Focusing on one or two specific issues

From the initial assessment a number of issues should emerge. Some of these may have been volunteered by the young person; others will have been perceived and shared by the helper. A summary is invaluable at this stage as a means of drawing together and identifying clearly the appropriate issues. Such a summary will lead quite naturally into focusing.

Focusing is:

> *The stage in the helping relationship where the helper and young person are able to choose the need/issue/problem to be dealt with in the next stage of the session.*

Such focusing lends a sense of direction and purpose to the remainder of the session. It consists of three main elements:

1 **Screening** Deciding which issues warrant time and effort in this interaction to enable us to agree and set priorities.
2 **Focusing** Explicitly agreeing with the young person which of these issues will form the basis of the remainder of the session.
3 **Clarification** Once an issue has been chosen for further exploration, it needs to be clarified so that the helper and young person know precisely what needs to be addressed. At this point, specific objectives can be set.

When focusing, beware of choosing the first/easiest, rather than the most pressing issue. Often young people will 'present' with topics. It is the helper's role to probe these topics with the young person to reveal any related issues that will require deeper exploration. The issue (or issues) chosen must be one that, if dealt with, will meet the young person's needs most effectively in the time available. Do not try to ignore those issues that you feel ill equipped to deal with. Be honest with the young person, try and work with them to address the issue, but be clear about the limitations of your professional help.

In focusing on the issue that gives most 'leverage' (Egan 2002), other issues may have to be ignored. Frequently, it is not possible to deal with all the relevant issues. One possible answer is to recognise this in a summary and acknowledge that you cannot cover all of them. The helper may deal with fundamental or relevant issues and point the young person in an appropriate direction in order to cope with others: either by making suggestions, or in more complex situations by referring on to, or advocating with, another agency or professional. Of course, where you are working with a young person who requires intensive support, you will both decide which issues can be dealt with, by whom and when, in the time you have contracted to work together.

The issue that is focused on, however, should form the theme for the remainder of the session. Together you can then go on to examine new perspectives, set appropriate goals for dealing with the issue, develop strategies for reaching goals and end with an agreed plan of action. One final note on focusing: it is perfectly acceptable and often a priority to renegotiate agreed issues as the session progresses. If further issues do emerge, it is essential that it is agreed which new issue is now forming the focus of the interview. In the case study below, what is the topic that the young person wants to focus on? Clearly you cannot spend time looking at all her presenting issues so what might be the central issue that you will both need to work on?

Case study: Neela – topics and issues in stage 1

Neela is cheerful, arriving early for her appointment. She enjoys her work in school although she says 'I'm not that clever.' It is easy to establish rapport and you have found out about her GCSE subjects, all of which she likes, and that she is studying hard for her mock exams.

Neela tells you she wants to stay in the sixth form, but also likes the college up the road. She goes on to say she enjoyed her work experience with a hairdresser and would like to work one day with children, or animals, or maybe in a travel agent (that's what her friend, Gemma, is going to do). Her mum says she's got to make her mind up but she doesn't know how. Her teacher said she should see you and you would 'sort her out'.

How are you going to focus?
What skills do you need?
What needs initial exploration at this point?
What are the topics and what is the underlying issue?

Neela wants your help, is friendly and there is much to talk about as she appears to have many interests. However, rather than divide the limited time into brief and therefore superficial explorations of all her interests, talking with a shared purpose would lead you to focus on the underlying issue rather than examine the topics. Why so many interests? Interests that are quite different. Who needs to make the decision? What are the external pressures on Neela, from Mum and the teacher, and how does she feel about this? What's the problem here – too many interests, or not knowing how to choose? How can Neela be helped to make a decision?

Common mistakes in Stage 1

We have looked at appropriate ways of working with and responding to young people in Stage 1. Set out below are some of the less helpful approaches which are sometimes taken:

- responses that imply condescension or manipulation;
- premature advice or premature discussion of action programmes;
- making inaccurate assumptions;
- running with the first topic rather than identifying issues related to needs;
- responses that indicate rejection of, or lack of respect for, the young person;

- responses involving premature confrontation (more about this later);
- responses that are patronising or placating;
- use of inaccurate reflections;
- use of clichés;
- responses that ignore the problem, change the subject or are otherwise irrelevant or judgemental.

It is impossible to overestimate the importance of getting this stage of the helping relationship right. In your desire to identify the topic or issue you may be tempted to rush through the early steps in Stage 1. Try to avoid doing this by taking the time needed for rapport building and clarification before 'getting' an agenda. On occasion, lack of time, or the organisation's need for information about young people, can place restraints on what you are trying to achieve. For instance you may need to check information and take notes. Do not let these get in the way of building rapport, as to a young person the notes can seem more important to you than what they have to say. Explaining what you are doing, and why, helps – and then put the notes to one side and give the young person your full attention. As you will be aware there are many things that need to be achieved in Stage 1, all of which are fundamental to the effectiveness or otherwise of the rest of the session. Unless the helper and the young person:

- have a shared understanding of the purpose and remit of the interaction;
- have a shared understanding of each other's role and contribution to the helping relationship;
- have begun to develop a rapport founded on respect and genuine interest – on which to base and generate a working relationship;
- have begun to address the young person's perceived needs;
- have attempted to set specific and achievable objectives for the session within the time and resources available

then it is highly likely that what follows will be ineffective, fail to meet the young person's real needs and fail to move them forward in a useful way. In addition, the young person is likely to go away not only with needs that have not been addressed, but also with a feeling of dissatisfaction or uncertainty about the value of the help they have just received. The case study below is not easy to 'solve'. Use it as a discussion exercise with colleagues. How can you help Joseph and demonstrate the core condition of 'unconditional positive regard'?

Case study: Joseph – sent for help and would rather be somewhere else

Joseph arrives at the centre to see someone, looking bored and resentful. You find his file and read in the notes that he left school before his sixteenth birthday after an incident involving drugs. There was a suggestion at the time that Joseph was using and selling drugs but this was not confirmed. Joseph is now 17 and is not in employment, education or training. You think he still lives at home but are not sure. You have done your best to build rapport and explained your role and the process, but Joseph is still not looking at you and yawns occasionally. You feel at this point the use of immediacy would be helpful – what are you going to say? (*Try to think of suitable ways of asking Joseph what is wrong*).

It worked! Joseph now starts talking and tells you that he is here because his mum 'has chucked him out because of his retail activity' (his words). He went to 'the social' but they said he had to come here and he doesn't see the point, he doesn't want a job, he needs somewhere to live. You know that you will need to discuss his future plans and you think it will be hard to get Joseph back after today. How are you going to meet his immediate needs and engage Joseph to work with you beyond today?

Immediacy is a direct challenging skill that can help to identify what is not working in the relationship between the helper and the young person. For example, saying to Joseph something like, 'I'm not sure what's happening here Joseph; I've probably not explained things properly. I'd like to help you, but at the moment I'm not sure what the problem is that I can help you with. What is it that I've missed?' In this example the helper takes the blame for the lack of rapport-building by asking the young person to 'put them right'. Once Joseph begins to work with you and the problem is identified, he will need to know that you (or a contact) will be able to deal with his immediate need. Having begun to build trust with him, he is more likely to think seeing you again is going to be worth a return visit.

Attention to all the key elements at this stage of the process, then, is vital. Time spent developing a good working relationship, a mutual understanding of the purpose and context, as well as some specific and achievable objectives, will ensure that the session is used purposefully and effectively – however much or little time is available. In addition, the young person's satisfaction is likely to be much greater. If you get Stage 1 right, the rest of the interaction (and in the case of Joseph, future work) will be built on a sound foundation.

In summary, negotiating the contract runs throughout Stage 1 as you work together towards mutual understanding of the purpose and process. Setting the agenda identifies the particular topics and issues you will move forward with into Stage 2.

Exercise: getting Stage 1 right

Getting the *process* of Stage 1 right is difficult and requires practice. You could try the following exercise with colleagues or even friends and family.

Choose a topic that is of interest to your interviewee, but steer clear of personal or emotional problems that you are not equipped to deal with. It could be a work or study decision, or a choice of holiday or another plan for the future. Using the skills outlined previously, concentrate on the steps in Stage 1, with the aim of clarifying the important issues to be discussed in the rest of the interview. You are aiming to negotiate the contract (ways of working together) and to clarify the agenda (focus on specific issues). Try to spend about ten minutes on this without deep exploration (just initial exploration), without finding solutions or suggesting action steps. If you hear yourself saying, 'Have you thought about . . .?', you've moved out of Stage 1! You could stop at the end of Stage 1 with a summary of the points raised and the agenda, but if you have achieved a purposeful agenda, keep going after the summary!

You will find that when you start to focus on the process you will forget to think about the skills and vice versa! This is frustrating but quite common; eventually the two will come together.

EFFECTIVE HELPING – THE PROCESS – STAGE 2

Stage 2 – preferred scenario (Egan 2002)
Developing issues and identifying goals (SIM)

Development is the central point of the work and Stage 2 is likely to be the stage where most time is spent. Everything prior to this is achieved to form a solid foundation for realistic development. As with the other stages of the process, identifying and responding to a young person's needs can be broken down into separate steps. That said, the work achieved in Stage 2 of the process is far less linear, and will often require you to re-negotiate the agenda to retain relevance and usefulness for the young person. When working with young people who require intensive support, you can still work towards a beginning, middle and end in each meeting, but it may be some time before you start or conclude this overall development and goal setting stage. Young people and helpers can get stuck in the process when external difficulties prevent progress. When this happens, returning to Stage 1, assessing the agenda and making adjustments, is sensible and purposeful for moving forward again.

Before we identify the steps for Stage 2, a reminder of the steps in Stage 1.

1   Assessing needs: helping the young person to tell their story.
2   Focusing: identifying issues to be addressed for the remainder of the work.

By going through these steps we:

- obtain a clear picture of the stage at which the young person is 'at' in the process of making decisions;
- can focus on agreed issues or needs;
- can help the young person to develop their thinking about their present position.

Challenging may help the young person to see the need to move on in their thinking and planning, but remember we need to 'earn the right to challenge'. *Goal setting* (the intended aim of Stage 2) completes this process by giving them something to aim at, a sense of purpose.

By 'allowing' the young person to tell their story in Stage 1, we have given them the 'space' to talk about what they already know before moving on to talk about things they, perhaps, do not yet know. The meaning of 'allowing' here is to ensure that time is allocated and made available for the story to be told: it does not imply permission or even encouragement, where the latter may be offered but not pursued. That said, some young people will find telling their story difficult and there are professional boundaries around how far you take this – your 'curiosity' must be relevant and it would not be collaborative to insist! However, ensuring time is available, and providing the young person with enough 'space' to tell their story, helps to build confidence and rapport. Having arrived at the development stage of the process (Stage 2), we can break this down into four steps. These are:

1   New perspectives – recognising other and new information that might affect the young person's choices.
2   Identification of possible goals.
3   Evaluation – helping the young person to be specific and to understand the consequences of their choices.
4   Choice and commitment – helping the young person to choose and commit themselves to action.

As said earlier, development is the central point or pivot upon which an effective collaboration turns. This is because it is the stage in the process when the young person is encouraged to look forward. Prior to this we have been defining issues; now we are attempting to generate solutions. Through developmental processes, we are helping the young person to identify what they wish to do and helping them to formulate these wishes into achievable goals.

Providing new perspectives

Most young people benefit from being moved beyond their own subjective understanding of their situation. In many cases, merely articulating their thoughts and focusing on relevant issues is unlikely to be sufficient. They need to be enabled to view their situation afresh: we can help them to gain a new perspective and new information. Often, old information and views need to be challenged: not discounted, but opened up to new possibilities. Having clearly defined the issues, we are beginning the process of moving the young person on. We are using our position as a 'skilled helper' to equip the young person to see things more clearly and to take control. Central to this step are the skills of sharing information and of challenging (discussed in the previous chapter).

One step at a time

Of course, with young people requiring intensive support the goals may be very small and immediate. In the early period of the working relationship it is unlikely that these goals are related to job choices or further education and training needs. There is a wide range of other goals that may need to be discussed and worked on, before the young person is ready to receive help with any vocational decision. This is part of the assessment activity of deciding 'where the client is at' in their current thinking and circumstances. That said, working on small and immediate goals brings a sense of achievement and is a learning process. Building on that success, future meetings work towards longer term goals, albeit at an appropriate pace within a time-bound working relationship.

Goals for young people requiring intensive support may include the development of a number of personal and social skills. In some situations the goals can be very practical, to cope with the 'here and now' before ideas for the future can be considered. For other young people short term goals may be broader and include information-finding ('finding out more about'), or self-assessment, before they can go on to identify more explicit goals. It is an obvious point, but goals are related to needs, and *how* you work collaboratively with the young person will depend on the amount of help they require, and you are able to give.

What makes goals relevant?

We can define goal setting as:

Deciding on what is to be done to help control the issue focused on.

What we are attempting to do is to generate a picture of what it would be like if the young person's issues were resolved and their needs were satisfied. To be useful, the goals you generate with the young person must be:

1 **Behavioural**, that is, concrete, specific and clear. A vaguely stated goal can only lead to vague action. In fact, it often leads to no action at all. For example, how often do we make resolutions to lose weight/eat 'healthy' foods/do more exercise? And how successful are these resolutions in most cases? Not very; we give up after a week or two usually because we do not make our goals specific. For instance, if we resolve to do more exercise, have we identified how much more exercise, when we are going to do it, what form the exercise will take, and so on? The what, how and when help us to (a) be specific, (b) know if the goal is realistic and (c) know when we have achieved it. So, if we are helping a young person to decide on a goal and plan of action, we need to check that we have specified what it is they are aiming to achieve by that action.

2 **Related to the issue.** If the previous steps in the work have not been undertaken effectively and clear issues have not been decided upon, then it is possible that goals will be established that are unrelated to the needs of the young person. Some helpers, in their eagerness to have the young person do something, subtly or overtly push them into setting goals that are not appropriate to them in their situation. In other words the goals are meaningful for the helper, but not for the young person in their context.

3 **Realistic**, that is, within the reach of the young person and in keeping with their abilities and interests. It is no good setting goals with a young person if they do not have, and cannot acquire, the skills needed to pursue the goals. On the other hand, some young people may need to be helped to realise the resources they do have. Helpers may challenge such young people to realise that the goals they had regarded as unattainable can be reached.

4 **Valued** by the young person. If they do not value a goal that seems to emerge from the processes of exploration and understanding, then encouraging them to pursue it can be 'whistling in the wind'. As above, be careful of trying to get a young person to set goals that would suit you if you were in their situation. It is one thing to challenge a young person to consider different goals and different options: it is another to try to get them to adopt what you value.

5 **Under the young person's control.** Sometimes certain goals cannot be achieved because things in the young person's environment prevent it – for example, their housing situation, their health, their family circumstances, a criminal record, substance dependency, the job or training market, their experiences at school, or other issues connected to the social and/or cultural context in which they operate. We need to be clear about what they can do on their own and what they will need help with.

6 **Verifiable.** One sign that goals are concrete and specific is when they can be verified in some way. Goals are meaningless if it is impossible to determine whether they have been achieved or not. Failure to establish verifiable goals can result in aimlessness. Helping young people to ask themselves how they will know that any given goal has been reached, is one way of challenging them to make their goals more concrete.

Once goals have been established, it is clear what is being aimed at. However, a client may not know how to reach this goal. This action-planning process forms Stage 3 of the model and is dealt with in detail in the next section. We must recognise that, in the process of setting goals, action steps by which these goals may be achieved often begin to emerge or suggest themselves, but it can be a mistake to pick the first one that seems to 'fit the bill'. In other words, although action will be discussed in Stage 2 of the work, specific action points (the what, the how, the where, the who else can help, the when and what next) are evaluated and discussed **in detail** in Stage 3. In the case study that follows, drawing on relevant skills and strategies, work through Stage 2 of the process to arrive at what you think would be the likely goals, but avoid detailing the action.

Case study: Rem – exploring a career idea

Imagine you are working with Rem who is 14 and is very keen on working with animals, 'probably as a vet'. From your discussion in Stage 1, you agreed an agenda of exploring the interest in work with animals and thinking about the options for work in this area. You also pick up on a number of issues that now need further clarification. These are 1) a school report that suggests attendance is a problem, 2) a lack of information on what is involved in being a vet and 3) some ambivalence about science subjects.

continued on next page

Stage 2

You want to avoid quizzing Rem with a stream of 'What do you know about . . .' or 'testing' questions. How are you going to explore Rem's interest, share information, challenge him and help him to arrive at achievable goals (not action yet!)? Try to avoid thinking about this in an abstract, third-person fashion, e.g. 'Well, you would need to . . .' Instead, write down what you would *actually do and say* – the words and strategies you would use to help Rem identify a goal or goals related to his interest. And, don't forget, the goal can be big, small, short term and/or long term.

At the exploration stage you will, of course, want to maintain rapport with Rem. He has told you of an interest in working with animals; the way to get a better understanding of this interest, and to introduce a discussion of the issues you identified in Stage 1, is to *stay with the interest*. If it is a real interest then there should be some energy behind the interest, in which case 'Tell me more about . . .' responses will encourage Rem to talk more. You would then continue with other open questions related to his responses (not the list of questions in your head), which then uncover the finer detail of his understanding. This approach will achieve the exploration, maintain rapport, demonstrate that you are interested in his perceptions and allow you both to share information and to reach a point when you can explore the issues or gaps in your combined knowledge. You will meet the aim of talking with a shared purpose. All the skills mentioned in the previous chapter will be useful but challenging is particularly useful in Stage 2. A back-up plan or an alternative to Rem's first idea may be useful but needs to be introduced at the right moment. The young person has a right to reject a back-up plan, but you have a duty to introduce the notion of alternatives so that they are aware of the range of options available before making a choice.

It's been said before, but when working with a young person over time you will re-negotiate the original agenda, in some cases at every meeting. This ensures that the work remains relevant for the young person and allows you both to assess the progress made, and the next steps for moving on. In extended work, goals are likely to change as a result of action taken or changed circumstances. For example, dropping out of a college course may seem like a negative step at first sight, but there may be positive reasons for this decision (a chance to travel or an unexpected job offer). As the work progresses, goals will need to be reviewed when the young person's ideas change: returning to the metaphor of the journey, horizons change for people when they are on the move.

EFFECTIVE HELPING – THE PROCESS – STAGE 3

Stage 3: getting there (Egan 2002)
Designing, planning and implementing action (SIM)

The function of this stage is to give the young person a clear idea about *how* they can achieve the goals set in Stage 2. Again, this stage has four steps and it is important to work through each step effectively, so that both the helper and young person have a clear sense of direction. The young person is then more likely to feel that their goals are attainable as a result of actions within their reach. Some of these actions may involve the helper, whilst others are things that the young person is quite able to do independently.

When young people come to a professional for help, their vision is often restricted and they can feel quite impotent. They may not be able to see that there are a variety of possible solutions or courses of action that they could take, and often they feel that they are in an either/or situation. The helper's task at this stage is to enable the young person to explore potential courses of action so that they can choose the most appropriate and, more importantly, feel that they can act upon decisions made to attain their goals.

The four steps within Stage 3 are:

1   Developing and evaluating strategies.
2   Choosing and planning a course of action.
3   Agreeing and taking action.
4   Conclusion.

We will look at each step in turn.

Developing strategies

Remember, the goal is where the young person wants to be. Strategies are the means of achieving the goal – how to get there. Strategies may be very simple or may be long and complicated, in which case it may be necessary to identify a series of sub-goals, each with its own set of strategies. This has been covered to some extent already in an earlier section of this chapter, but is linked here, explicitly, to this stage of the helping process.

Many young people know what they want, but have no real idea how to achieve it, so may try the first thing that comes to mind, without being clear about how effective the action is likely to be in achieving their goals. The role of the helper is to enable the young person to consider a range of possibilities, and to identify those that are most likely to work for them.

A 'thought shower' of different ways of reaching a goal can help: it can lead to a wider choice, and some of the less obvious strategies generated may be more appropriate and effective. The list itself may stimulate the young person's imagination and help them to think of further possibilities.

It is essential to be creative during this process. A young person may need help and encouragement with this. The concept of divergent thinking can be useful here; this involves getting away from the 'one right answer' approach (convergent thinking). Several important rules help to make the thought shower technique work:

- **Suspend judgement**   Do not let the young person be critical of the strategies being generated, and do not criticise them yourself.
- **Let yourself go**   Encourage the young person to include even the wildest possibilities, as they can always be left out later but may include elements that are practical.
- **Encourage quantity**   The more alternatives there are, the better chance of finding useful strategies.
- **Piggyback**   Encourage the young person to add on to the strategies already generated.
- **Clarify items**   Getting the young person to clarify points can lead to new possibilities.
- **Prompts**   Once goals have been identified, you can use prompts to help a young person identify strategies, for example:

  - People: who can help the young person achieve the goal?
  - Models: does the young person know anyone who does what they want to do?
  - Places: where to go.
  - Things: what else will help?
  - Skills: which skills the young person already has that will help.

Once started, the list of possibilities often appears endless. Generating strategies is an important step in helping young people to consider alternatives and, in turn, helps them to feel that there is a solution, or even a range of solutions. The thought shower process often releases a great deal of creativity and it is surprising how often a suggestion, which previously would have been discounted immediately as impossible, leads to some action when it is considered in this way. It can also be fun and helps to retain the engagement of the young person.

The next step is to evaluate the results of the thought shower.

Choosing and planning courses of action

Once the strategies have been identified, it is necessary to choose those that are most appropriate. Strategies to achieve goals must have certain characteristics. They must be **SMART**:

- specific;
- measurable or verifiable;
- attainable;
- realistic;
- timebound;

and also be:

- owned by the young person;
- valued by the young person.

You will recognise some of these points from Stage 2.

To choose and plan action, there are various activities the helper can use to assist the young person to evaluate the strategies identified in the thought shower. Egan (2002) discusses such activities in detail, and it is worth looking at a variety of methods to evaluate strategies with young people, in order to have a range of methods to choose from. Some will be more appropriate than others: for different young people and their goals. We have considered many already in chapter 6. We will look at one method again, here, that can be used for both goal setting and evaluating possible courses of action.

Force-field analysis

Force-field analysis is particularly effective at this stage of the process. The aim of this method is to consider the elements (forces) that hinder an option and the elements that will facilitate action. Using this method, the young person is able to assess how useful or otherwise the strategy is in helping them towards their goal.

Here is a simple example: Stage 3 moving to action

You are working with Alex, whose eventual goal is to 'one day' get a job working with young children. Together you have identified a range of strategies that might facilitate this, including various information finding techniques and possible routes into the work. Alex needs help in evaluating the possible routes to assess which one will suit best. You agree to evaluate the route of going to college to do a vocational course, using force-field analysis. A word of caution at this point: avoid using the technical term as it can be off-putting – suggesting that you look at the pros and cons of an idea is likely to be more helpful.

continued on next page

To evaluate the possible option of going to college to take a vocational course, you use the thought shower technique to identify a range of possible restraints:

- lack of money;
- need for parental support which is doubtful at present;
- anxiety about failing, possibly wasting two years;
- uncertainty about a commitment to two more years of education;
- an unfamiliar place.

And you also identify possible facilitating forces:

- strong motivation to work with children;
- extra time to find out more before committing self to job;
- great interest in work experience opportunities;
- a close friend is also interested in going to college;
- the chance to make new friends.

The next step is to help Alex to check whether all the restraints and facilitating forces are applicable, particularly the restraining forces, so that they are prepared for any difficulties. Working through the forces in this way will help Alex not only to evaluate the feasibility of a course of action, but also to choose which is most suitable for them.

Now, continue the story – what do you think would be SMART action points for Alex? Try to think this through as the helper and as Alex.

In going through the options a young person will often begin to favour one or more courses of action that they feel comfortable with. This will facilitate the likelihood of action and ultimate success in the achievement of goals. You can apply force-field analysis to a number of situations, not just for vocational outcomes, so that the young person can compare the feasibility of alternatives. Even young people for whom a training, education or career choice may have to be set aside for the present in the face of more immediate needs, may still have choices where the available options and action steps need to be evaluated. However, immediate needs should not stop us from considering action for the future. It is worth considering that when faced with a range of multiple issues to be resolved, an exploration of a different future, related to a 'dream' career, can energise a young person to look forward beyond what at present may seem like insurmountable problems.

Agreeing and taking action

For many young people it will be enough for the helper to work with them through the exploration and decision making phases – they will then feel able to go ahead with the action steps on their own. In other cases, the young person and helper will agree that they both need to take some action and, in some cases, the young person will require support in implementing the action that they have chosen to undertake.

Many young people will benefit from help in formulating an action plan. This can help them to break down tasks into small steps that they feel are achievable. Action plans need to be specific and realistic, and allow a reasonable time frame for the achievement of action and goals.

Some young people will require additional support such as advocacy (as discussed on page 35), for instance initiating a contact with an employer, arranging a personal interview with a college tutor or liaising with a health or social worker. Support for a young person can also take the form of meeting again, within a specified period, to review the young person's progress in implementing the agreed action. You would then review options for further action in the light of outcomes from the action agreed.

WARNING!

Stage 3 is about evaluating and planning action, *not* merely writing an action plan. Without proper evaluation of the action steps to achieve goals, any agreed action is likely to be imposed on the young person by the helper. If the action plan is not negotiated and the purpose not shared, then the agreement is compliant with the helper's ideas and is unlikely to be 'owned' and 'actioned' by the young person.

Exercise: listening to the psychological message

It is important throughout the meeting to attend to body language and to listen attentively, but near the end of the session this sometimes gets forgotten. When discussing action steps, it is also important to listen to the psychological message that underlies the apparent affirmative answer. What do you think the psychological message might be in the following responses from a young person to suggested action; suggested by the helper?

'Well, I could try.'
'I could ask my teacher.'

continued on next page

'I might go to the open day.'
'I'll see if I can contact that person.'

If the helper's response is 'Good, that's settled then' what do you think has not been 'heard' here? What needs to be clarified or challenged, and how would you do this in a helpful way? Again, as in the exercise with Rem, think of the actual words you could use.

To help the young person to evaluate action steps, and to ensure that the agreed action is SMART for them, you are likely to use challenging skills. For example, 'When you say you will try, I am picking up that it could be difficult. Why might that be the case?'; 'We've said you could ask your teacher. How easy would that be for you?'; 'You say you might go to the open day. What would stop you going?'; 'What would help you, or stop you, making contact with that person?' The answers will reveal what may be a worrying issue for the young person that you had not considered, but is easily resolved: for instance in the third example, 'I don't know where the college is'.

Conclusion

Good beginnings are very important. At the beginning of the helping relationship it is important to set the scene, clarify and agree the purpose, create a rapport with the young person and decide where to begin. Likewise, endings are important, whether the ending is the conclusion of a series of sessions, where the young person and helper work together, or a one-off meeting when the young person is ready to progress and act on their own as a result of the single session.

Endings help to 'wrap things up' and may be a point at which it is appropriate to undertake some final clarification or checking out. For example, clarifying that the young person is clear about 'where they have got to' as a result of the session and their next steps, or checking that they feel at ease with what has been agreed. The conclusion is also the point of leave-taking, goodbye or 'see you again soon'. The social skills required for greetings are needed here too, so that the conclusion is clear and smooth, as well as obvious to both the helper and the young person. Abrupt conclusions can leave the young person feeling disconcerted, or even rejected, and an inadequate conclusion can diminish or undermine the feeling of something valuable achieved. Time taken over a conclusion is more likely to help both the young person and the helper to feel positive when a session ends. It is important to avoid the closed, 'Was that helpful?' Asking the young person 'What do you think we've achieved today?' or 'How has that helped?' will give you an evaluative statement and may reveal an issue that was not covered but can be discussed next time.

With the conclusion, the helping process is brought to an end. In using the Single Interaction Model, you will be working towards the position where both the young person and you, the helper, feel that progress has been made, and that the young person is now ready to move on. In long term work, when you are aware that you and the young person are meeting for the last time, in the conclusion you will reflect on the work achieved – the journey or 'distance travelled' – to celebrate the achievements the young person has made.

Before concluding this chapter, an exercise follows to help you to contextualise the model for aspects of your work. If you do not have this level of experience as yet, this could be a group activity, or an exercise that you undertake with a colleague or your mentor, based on an observation of practice.

The Single Interaction Model in practice

Identify two or three young people you have worked with, or are working with, that 'fit' into the engagement model described in figures 2.2 and 2.4 (pages 16 and 21). For each young person **tell the story** of the help they received, with reference to the three-stage SIM, as outlined in figures 2.1 and 2.3.

Think about how the model fits with this work:

- Was there a clear beginning, middle and end in each meeting?
- How do you negotiate a contract?
- What was the agenda?
- What was the issue or issues that needed exploring?
- How were these identified?
- What were the goals as a result of the helping?
- How was action discussed?
- What was agreed?
- What happened next?

Now, if appropriate, *retell the story* for one of the examples and make it a better story, using your understanding of the model. If you changed the story, to make it a better story with a more positive outcome, reflect on how the process, the skills and strategies that you introduced, worked to re-frame the work. This reflection may help you to think about the areas you wish to develop further.

A final word

In this chapter we have looked at each stage of the Single Interaction Model and the steps within each stage. In practice the work is rarely this linear, but the structure, once familiar, will help you and your young person to recognise where you are in the helping process.

The book has focused on the various elements in the process of developing helping relationships with young people. We have explored the context of working with young people, and we have explained how the interpersonal skills we use in our everyday lives can be used effectively in helping relationships. The knowledge of how things work can enable us to enhance our practice for the benefit of the young people we work with.

We have presented a Single Interaction Model, which is intended to provide a sound basis for professional helpers working with young people. For work with those young people who require intensive support, this Single Interaction Model can be sited within the larger Egan framework, to acknowledge the ongoing nature of the relationship. However, in working towards positive outcomes, at whatever stage, all interactions can follow a beginning, middle and end structure. The structure provides a learning process that assists both the helper and the young person to move on. For the practitioner it provides a framework onto which you will build your own model reflecting your knowledge, experience and engagement as you continue to develop and enhance your professional practice. We hope that the structure will enhance your ability to engage effectively with young people: to achieve talking with a shared purpose in those relationships.

We have also referred to other models and approaches which we hope you will investigate further: there are many more that we have been unable to find space to mention. Additional reading will provide you with further tools to think and act with. Skilled helpers have a responsibility to develop 'knowledgeable practice' beyond their initial practical knowledge: young people deserve no less.

Annotated reading list

These texts have been chosen to provide additional background to the integrated approach covered in *Providing Support to Young People*. It is in no way an exhaustive list, and practitioners may well find that they have other 'favourites' that they prefer to use. In terms of the 'knowledgeable practice' mentioned earlier, this is fine! These are the books which have influenced the development of the model, or which we have found particularly useful for working with young people.

Coleman, J.C. and Hendry, L.B. (1999) *The Nature of Adolescence*, 3rd edn, London and New York: Routledge.

- A thorough exploration of the nature of young people's lives, this book is particularly useful in helping us to understand the complexity and uncertainty faced by many young people.

Culley, S. and Bond, T. (2004) *Integrative Counselling Skills in Action*, 2nd edn, London: Sage.

- This is a very useful foundation text, and the style of writing is very accessible. It will be of especial interest to helpers whose practice is with young people with more intensive support needs, and who draw extensively on counselling approaches.

Egan, G. (2002) *The Skilled Helper: A Problem-Management and Opportunity-Development Approach to Helping*, 7th edn, Pacific Grove, California: Brooks/Cole.

- This book provides a very detailed look at a three-stage approach to counselling, which has formed a large part of the background to the integrated model presented here. It is very useful as a reference, to use in relation to specific issues concerning process in an interview and the use of skills in helping young people. It is particularly useful once you have gained more experience working with young people.

Fouad, N.A. and Bingam, R.P. (1995) 'Career counselling with racial and ethnic minorities', in W.B. Walsh and S.H. Osipow (eds.) *Handbook of Vocational Psychology: Theory, Research and Practice*, Mahwah, New Jersey: Lawrence Erlbaum Associates.

- Fouad and Bingam's work recognises the need to place guidance within a multicultural context and offers a model for structuring such work. Although focused on career guidance, the principles can be applied to providing wider support for young people.

Kidd, J.M. (2006) *Understanding Career Counselling: Theory, Research and Practice*, London: Sage.

- This book brings together theory, research and practice in relation to career counselling. The first part will be particularly relevant to those involved in career guidance practice, as it links career theory to practice. The second part is of more general relevance and looks at counselling skills, tools and techniques.

Nelson-Jones, R. (2005) *Practical Counselling and Helping Skills*, 5th edn, London: Cassell.

- As the title suggests, this is a very practical look at the skills used in helping clients. Though it also has counselling as its starting point, it is relevant to the youth support context. It offers an alternative to Egan in the 'lifeskills counselling model' presented.

O'Connell, B. (1998) *Solution Focused Brief Therapy*, London: Sage.

- This book gives a comprehensive introduction to SFBT from the foremost writer of the approach in the UK. Alongside an exploration of theory that informs solution focused work, there are detailed examples of using the approach in practice.

Rogers, C.R. (1951) *Client-Centred Therapy*, London: Constable.
Rogers, C.R. (2004) *On Becoming a Person*, London: Constable.

- Fundamental texts for humanistic counselling. They are very much rooted in the therapeutic background, but have much to offer professional helping: the books are seminal. The second was originally published in the USA in 1961 – this is the new London edition.

Rollnick, S. and Miller, W.R. (1995) 'What is motivational interviewing?' *Behavioural and Cognitive Psychotherapy*, 23, pp. 325–334. Online. Available at www.motivationalinterview.org (accessed 22 April 2005).

- Rollnick and Miller define motivational interviewing as both directive, and client-centred. It aims to work towards behaviour change by helping clients to explore and resolve areas in their thinking about the future that they are ambivalent or indecisive about. The approach is more focused and goal-directed than many counselling models. Motivational interviewing can be helpful where young people are 'stuck' and finding it difficult to move forward, or where there are many problems or issues to be resolved. We have used this 1995 text as our starting point for this book, but an update on their work can be found in Miller, W.R. and Rollnick, S. (2002) *Motivational Interviewing: Preparing People for Change*, 2nd edn, New York: Guildford Press.

Winslade, J. and Monk, G. (1999) *Narrative Counseling in Schools*, Thousand Oaks, California: Corwin Press Inc.

- With just 124 pages of text this is accessible, concise and, through case study examples, demonstrates how a 'bad' story can be changed into a 'good' story via solution focused and narrative work. The authors also offer a guide through many of the techniques that have been introduced in *Providing Support to Young People*. Although based on school counselling the application is wider and can be applied to other situations where 'traditional' approaches are found to be less effective. It is suitable for both the novice and experienced practitioner.

References

Bassot, B. (2003) 'Towards a situated learning theory for careers education and guidance', *Career Research and Development, The NICEC Journal*, No. 10, Winter, pp. 10–14.

Bateman, N. (1995) *Advocacy Skills: A Handbook for Human Service Professionals*, Aldershot and Vermont: Arena Ashgate Publishing Limited.

Berne, E. (1968) *Games People Play: The Psychology of Human Relationships*, St Ives: Penguin.

Besley, A.C. (2002) *Counselling Youth: Foucault, Power and the Ethics Of Subjectivity*, Westport, Connecticut: Praeger.

Bimrose, J. (1996) 'Multiculturalism', in R. Bayne, I. Horton and J. Bimrose (eds), *New Directions in Counselling*, London: Routledge, pp. 237–246.

Brown, H. (2003) *Safe Connexions: Protection of Young People within the Connexions Service*, Canterbury Christ Church University: Occasional Paper, Centre for Career and Personal Development.

Chambers Dictionary (1988) 7th edn, London: Chambers.

COIC/CSNU (2001) *A Little Book of Evaluation*, Nottingham: Department for Education and Skills/CSNU. Online. Available at www.connexions.gov.uk/partnerships/pulications/uploads/cp/ACF2D35.pdf.

Coleman, J.C., and Hendry, L. B. (1999) *The Nature of Adolescence*, 4th edn, London and New York: Routledge.

CSNU (Connexions Service National Unit) (2003) *Code of Practice for Connexions Personal Advisers*, Reference Number CXP 124, Moorfoot, Sheffield: CSNU, Department for Education and Skills.

Corfield, R. (1995) *The Careers Adviser's Guide: How to Give Practical Job Search Advice to Clients*, London: Kogan Page.

Culley, S. and Bond, T. (2004) *Integrative Counselling Skills in Action*, 2nd edn, London: Sage.

Daniels, D. and Jenkins, P. (2000) *Therapy with Children: Children's Rights, Confidentiality and the Law*, London: Sage.

DfES (Department for Education and Skills) (2003) *Every Child Matters, cm 5860*. Online. Available at www.everychildmatters.gov.uk (accessed 1 February 2006).

—— (2005) *Youth Matters, cm6629*, Norwich: Her Majesty's Stationery Office.

Dewson, S., Eccles, J., Tackey, N.D. and Jackson, A. (2000) *Guide to Measuring Soft Outcomes and Distance Travelled*, Brighton: Institute of Employment Studies for Department of Education and Employment.

Edwards, R. (1998) 'Mapping, locating and translating: a discursive approach to professional development', *Studies in Continuing Education*, 20(1), pp. 23–38.

Egan, G. (2002) *The Skilled Helper: A Problem-Management and Opportunity-Development Approach to Helping*, 7th edn, Pacific Grove, California: Brooks/Cole.

Epston, D. (1989).*Collected Papers*, Adelaide: Dulwich Centre.

Fielding, A.J. (1999) 'Where do we go from here?', ICG Occasional Paper, *Constructing Models of Guidance for the Millennium*, Stourbridge: Institute of Career Guidance, pp. 29–37.

Fouad, N.A. and Bingam, R.P. (1995) 'Career counselling with racial and ethnic minorities', in W.B. Walsh and S.H. Osipow (eds) *Handbook of Vocational Psychology: Theory, Research and Practice*, Mahwah, New Jersey: Lawrence Erlbaum Associates.

Gothard, B., Mignot, P., Offer, M. and Ruff, M. (2001) *Careers Guidance in Context*, London: Sage Publications.

Honey, P. and Mumford, A. (1992) *The Manual of Learning Styles*, 3rd edn, Maidenhead: Peter Honey.

Jayasinghe, M. (2001) *Counselling in Careers Guidance*, Buckingham: OU Press.

Johnson, D.W. and Johnson, F.P. (1994) *Joining Together: Group Theory and Group Skills*, Needham Heights, Massachusetts: Allyn and Bacon.

Kidd, J.M. (1996) 'The career counselling interview', in A.G. Watts, B. Law, J. Killeen, J.M. Kidd, and R. Hawthorn (eds) *Rethinking Careers Education and Guidance: Theory, Policy and Practice*, London: Routledge, pp. 189–209.

—— (2006) *Understanding Career Counselling: Theory, Research and Practice*, London: Sage.

Killeen, J. (1996) 'Evaluation', in A.G. Watts, B. Law, J. Killeen, J.M. Kidd and R. Hawthorn (eds) *Rethinking Careers Education and Guidance: Theory, Policy and Practice*, London: Routledge, pp. 331–348.

Law, B. (1996) 'A career-learning theory', in A.G. Watts, B. Law, J. Killeen, J.M. Kidd and R. Hawthorn (eds) *Rethinking Careers Education and Guidance: Theory, Policy and Practice*, London: Routledge, pp. 46–71.

McLeod, J. (1997) *Narrative and Psychotherapy*, London: Sage.

Maslow, A.H. (1987) *Motivation and Personality*, 3rd edn, New York: Longman.

Miller, W.R. and Rollnick, S. (2002) *Motivational Interviewing: Preparing People for Change*, 2nd edn, New York: Guildford Press.

Mulvey, M.R. (2002) 'Ethical practice in guidance: do the right thing', in K. Roberts (ed.) *Constructing the Future: Social Inclusion, Policy and Practice*, Stourbridge: Institute of Career Guidance, pp. 79–89.

Nelson-Jones, R. (2005) *Practical Counselling and Helping Skills: Text and Exercises for the Lifeskills Counselling Model*, 5th edn, London: Sage Publications.

O'Connell, B. (2001) *Solution-Focused Stress Counselling*, London: Continuum Books.

Reid, H.L. (2002) 'Are you sitting comfortably? Stories and the usefulness of narrative approaches', in K. Roberts (ed.) *Constructing the Future: Social Inclusion, Policy and Practice*, Stourbridge: Institute of Career Guidance, pp. 51–66.

—— (2004) 'Jiminy Cricket on my shoulder: ethical watchfulness and the place of support and supervision for personal advisers', in H.L. Reid and J. Bimrose (eds) *Career Guidance, Constructing the Future: Reflection on Practice*, Stourbridge: Institute of Career Guidance, pp. 39–54.

—— (2005) 'Beyond the toolbox: integrating multicultural principles into a career guidance intervention model', in B. Irving and B. Malik (eds) *Critical Reflections on Career Education and Guidance: Promoting Social Justice within a Global Economy*, London: Routledge, pp. 172–185.

—— (2006) 'Introduction – constructing the future: transforming career guidance', in H.L. Reid and J. Bimrose (eds) *Constructing the Future: Transforming Career Guidance*, Stourbridge: Institute of Career Guidance.

Reid, H.L. and Westergaard, J. (2006) *Providing Support and Supervision: An Introduction for Professionals Working with Young People*, London: Routledge.

Rogers, C.R. (1951) *Client-Centred Therapy*, London: Constable.

Rogers, C.R. (1961) *On Becoming a Person*, Boston: Houghton Mifflin.

Rogers, C.R. (2004) *On Becoming a Person*, London: Constable.

Rollnick, S. and Miller, W.R. (1995) 'What is motivational interviewing?' *Behavioural and Cognitive Psychotherapy*, 23, pp. 325–334. Online. Available at www.motivationalinterview.org (accessed 22 April 2005).

Schon, D. (1983) *The Reflective Practitioner: How Professionals Think in Action*, London: Temple Smith.

SEU (Social Exclusion Unit) (1999) *Bridging the Gap: New Opportunities for 16–18 Year Olds Not in Education, Employment or Training*, London: Stationery Office.

Sue, D.W., Allen, E.I. and Pederson, P.B. (1996) *A Theory of Multicultural Counseling and Therapy*, Pacific Grove, California: Brooks/Cole.

UDACE (Unit for the Development of Adult and Continuing Education) (1986) *The Challenge of Change*, London: UDACE.

Watts, A.G. (2006) 'Disconnecting Connexions', in H.L. Reid (ed.) *Re-positioning Careers Education and Guidance*, Occasional Paper, Centre for Career and Personal Development, Canterbury Christ Church University, pp. 1–8.

Westergaard, J. (2003) 'Counselling and the PA role – are these connected?' *British Journal of Guidance and Counselling*, 31(2), pp. 241–250.

White, M. and Epston, D. (1990) *Narrative Means to Therapeutic Ends*, Adelaide: Dulwich Centre.

Winslade, J. and Monk, G. (1999) *Narrative Counseling in Schools*, Thousand Oaks, California: Corwin Press Inc.

Index